The History of Medicine in Jerusalem

Zohar Amar

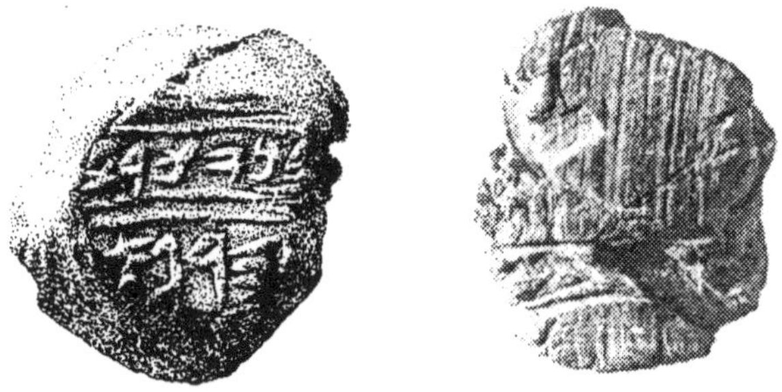

BAR International Series 1032

2002

Published in 2016 by
BAR Publishing, Oxford

BAR International Series 1032

The History of Medicine in Jerusalem

ISBN 978 1 84171 412 7

BAR Publishing is the trading name of British Archaeological Reports (Oxford) Ltd. British Archaeological Reports was first incorporated in 1974 to publish the BAR Series, International and British. In 1992 Hadrian Books Ltd became part of the BAR group. This volume was originally published by Archaeopress in conjunction with British Archaeological Reports (Oxford) Ltd / Hadrian Books Ltd, the Series principal publisher, in 2002. This present volume is published by BAR Publishing, 2016.

Printed in England

BAR
PUBLISHING

BAR titles are available from:

BAR Publishing
122 Banbury Rd, Oxford, OX2 7BP, UK
EMAIL info@barpublishing.com
PHONE +44 (0)1865 310431
FAX +44 (0)1865 316916
www.barpublishing.com

Dedicated

To my wife Tamar
and to our children
Shakéd, Yadin, Tzur, Mevasseret, and Matanya

Table of Contents

"There are ten things that God will renew in the days to come...the second is "taking living water out of Jerusalem and curing everyone who is sick" (Shemot Rabba 15:21).

Preface

This work joins a long series of studies conducted in recent years at the Department for Land of Israel Studies at Bar-Ilan University in the Unit for the History of Medicine in Ancient Times. Since the field of study is extensive, the special focus of this treatise is the study of medicine in Greater Jerusalem, but it may serve as a faithful reflection of the nature of medicine and the changes it underwent throughout Israel and Syria in ancient times.

This study is based primarily on historical sources of uneven quantity and quality; there are few direct accounts from Biblical times in comparison with information from later periods. In effect, the information from all of the historical periods is sporadic, which frequently makes it difficult to sketch an authentic, comprehensive representation and limits the possibilities of drawing categorical conclusions. Due to these constraints, we have not presumed to present a thorough survey of medicine in Jerusalem during Biblical times and the Second Temple period, and instead have contented ourselves with citing some of the information available on that subject. Accordingly the main thrust of the essay will focus on a chronological interval of approximately one thousand years, beginning with the Byzantine period, through the Middle Ages and into modern times.

The first part of the book consists of a short history of medicine in Jerusalem from various historical aspects, followed by an evaluation of the physicians, their status, professional training, etc. The second part presents a list of physicians who were active in Jerusalem between the 10th-18th centuries which is the focus of this study.

Throughout history Jerusalem was ruled by diverse nations and cultures who influenced medicine in the city in one form or another. Thus, for example, it is of considerable importance to examine the accounts of medicine in Jerusalem in light of the circumstances in the various cultural centers which controlled Jerusalem such as Mesopotamia, Egypt, Greece, and Rome, and later the Arabs and Ottomans. Without ignoring these centers of influence the authors focused first and foremost on the sources that relate directly to Jerusalem – which is the heart of this study. In addition to the historical sources, we will present the archeological findings that were uncovered in Jerusalem, beginning with the first results of the intensive archeological research taking place in the city in recent generations. The object of this study is to collect as much information as possible on medicine in Jerusalem through the centuries, for though it is a city which has stimulated an enormous body of research literature and is still a lodestone for scholars from diverse fields of interest, the aspect of medicine has been almost ignored (except for modern times). Furthermore, a large part of the written sources for this study (Jewish law sources and modern research literature) have been available until now only in Hebrew, making them inaccessible to most readers, and thus the importance of presenting these sources here for the first time in English.

The object of the study was to show that there was extensive medical activity in the city of Jerusalem over the generations, both because of its centrality to the religions of many nations and because of political interests. This is particularly true of the transition phase between the Byzantine Period and the Middle Ages. A fascinating chapter in the history of medicine in Jerusalem was written during the period of Crusader control of the city, apropos the extensive documentation of the Hospitallers' activity in their 'house of the sick'. It seems that the craft of medicine in Jerusalem achieved its peak during the Ayyubid Period. Beginning in the Mamluk Period, medicine began to suffer a decline, part of the overall trend that characterized the entire Far East. During the Ottoman Period we are witness to the first appearances of European medicine in Jerusalem, due in no small part to the fact that Jews migrated from the European continent to Jerusalem. However, there was no substantial change in the standard of medicine until the second half of the nineteenth century. This study therefore offers an opportunity to obtain an insight into the circuitous progress of medical tradition and its shift from east to west and from the ancient period to the modern.

Special thanks are in order to Professor Joshua Schwartz who heads the Jerusalem Project of the G.C. Foundation who came up with the idea for this study and Dr. Efraim Lev, my good friend and partner in the study of the history of medicine. Many thanks to Shifra Blass who labored over the translation of the book from Hebrew to English under sometimes difficult circumstances, and did so pleasantly and patiently. I would like to thank Mr. David Davison, Director of Archeopress Publishers who was sympathetic to this study and brought it to publication. And last but never least, I would like to thank my family, my wife Tamar and our five children: Shakéd, Yadin, Tzur, Mevasseret, and Matanya to whom this study is dedicated.

The author

PART ONE

Chapter One

Some information about medicine during Biblical times

There are a number of written accounts and archaeological documentation of medicine during the First Temple Period with the Bible constituting the principle source of information. The first accounts of medicine appear during the period of the Judean kings for whom Jerusalem served as their capital. It is only natural that the Biblical text describes the reality prevalent among the elite, which makes it difficult for us to learn of the character and status of medical science among the general population.

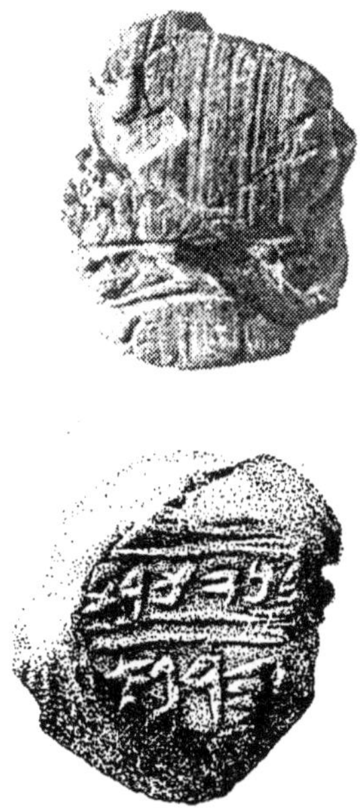

[לטבשלם]
בן זכר
הרפא

Figure 1: Bulla from the City of David with the inscription "le-Tavshalem ben Zachar Harofe" (early 6th century BCE)

Being a physician was a profession[1] recognized in Jerusalem and evidence of this is a bulla from the early 6th century B.C.E. uncovered in the City of David with the inscription: 'לטבשלם בן זכר הרפא' [le-Tavshalem ben Zachar Harofe] [Fig. 1].[2] It seems that the physician le-Tavshalem was a descendant of a distinguished family whose sons were physicians. The reference is to a prominent personality who must have held a position in the government. In ancient Egypt and Mesopotamia, too, there were physicians who held official positions.[3] With regard to King Asa there is mention of the 'רפאים' [physicians] he consulted during his illness:

"And Asa in the thirty-ninth year of his reign was diseased in his feet until his disease became severe; yet in his disease he did not seek the Lord but the physicians. And Asa slept with his fathers and died in the forty-first year of his reign. And they buried him in his own tomb, which he had made for himself in the city of

---

[1] For more on the term 'rophe" [physician], see: Preuss, pp. 11, 18-19.
[2] Shiloh, pp. 73-87; Shoham, pp. 151-175; Avigad & Sass, p. 177.
[3] Leibowitz, pp. 408-410.

David, and laid him on a bier which was filled with sweet odors and divers kinds of spices prepared by the perfumer's art, and they made a very great burning for him".[4]

It is clear from this source that it was professional physicians who served the kings, and it is not clear whether the common folk enjoyed their services as well. In any case, from this text there is nothing to be learned that suggests a negative attitude toward the medical profession. It appears that the text is specifically critical of Asa who was content to rely on conventional medicine and did not pray for divine healing. According to the perception expressed by this text, the real physician is God and mortal physicians are merely his agents. The person who observes the commandments of the Lord is guaranteed a complete recovery.[5] This point is very important since medicine in Jerusalem during the Temple period was not divorced from the religious aspect. Alongside of conventional medicine, the sick, especially those who suffered from incurable diseases, apparently used to make pilgrimages to the Temple and pray to be healed. We learn this from the prayer of King Solomon during the inauguration of the Temple.[6] In contrast, the Bible prominently records the punishment of those who did not follow the path divinely ordered. This was the punishment of the Judean king Yehoram in consequence of his evil deeds:

"And after all this the Lord smote him in his bowels with an incurable disease. And it came to pass that in process of time, after the end of two years, his bowels came out by reason of his sickness; so he died in great agony."[7]

Another story that demonstrates the Bible's approach is the case of the terminal illness of King Hezekiah who suffered from boils. Healing was effected miraculously by means of the prophet, and this was made public when the king went up to the house of the Lord:

"In those days Hezekiah fell mortally sick. And the prophet Isaiah the son of Amoz came to him and said, Thus says the Lord, Set they house in order, for thou shalt die, and not live. Then he turned his face to the wall, and prayed to the Lord, saying, I beseech thee O Lord remember now how I have walked before thee…and it came to pass that the word of the Lord came to him (through the prophet Isaiah) saying… I have heard thy prayer, I have seen thy tears: behold, I will heal you. On the third day thou shalt go up to the house of the Lord."[8]

Another reference that is connected with this story is the cure used in King Hezekiah's illness:

---

[4] 2 Ch., 16: 12-14. Cf: 2 Ch. 21:19, Jer. 34:5; T. Shabat , 7:18.
[5] See i.e. Ex. 15:26; 23:25; Prv. 3:7-8.
[6] 1 Kings 8:37; 2 Ch. 6:28.
[7] 2 Ch. 21:18-19.
[8] 2 Kings 20:1-5.

"And Isaiah said: Take a cake of figs. And they took and laid it on the festering place and he recovered."[9] The rabbinic sages amplify the miraculous cure and contend that this was "a miracle within a miracle" since figs, just like the sickness of boils "consume the flesh",[10] in other words, the method of cure employed was one that recalls the homeopathic method. However, based on the simple interpretation of the text it would seem that one may learn that treatment with cakes of figs was part of the conventional method using in curing boils in those times. A similar treatment using figs against various skin diseases is known to us from traditional medicine in the Near East.[11]

In Biblical times there was also a local folk medicine which involved a partial element of magic. Faint traces of this may be seen in findings discovered in a large cave dated to the eighth century B.C.E. which was found on the fringes of the city of David near the Gihon Spring. The cave contained, among others, many clay pots and residues of foodstuffs, and other findings which indicate that this was neither a burial cave nor a regular cave for dwelling. The researchers conjectured that it might have been a shrine belonging to a folk healer or a wise (wo)man who served as a kind of healer and to whom people turned to for healing from sickness, to achieve fertility, etc. [12] Some scholars believe that the רפאים 'Rephaim'[13] mentioned in the Bible dealt with effecting cures of the sick through magic (by means of water) and their name was derived from the verb 'רפא' which means "to heal". In their opinion, The Valley of the Rephaim[14] (or the Valley of the Healers) surrounding Jerusalem was named after these healers.[15]

The Bible differentiates between a cure sent by God through a miracle and a cure through magic, which it rejects out of hand. There is a well-known Biblical story about the "brass serpent" which Moses created at the command of God and which was used to bring about the plague of venomous snakes which cost the people many casualties.[16] Here, too, one may see in this act a symbol of a miracle within a miracle, using the plague itself to remove the plague. According to Biblical tradition, the brass serpent was preserved in the First Temple in Jerusalem until the time of Hezekiah. Over time it became a kind of fetish or cult object of idolatry, until King Hezekiah was forced to grind it down and destroy it.[17] This serpent was undoubtedly also perceived by some of the people as an object to which they attributed unique healing properties. Another example which evokes the brass serpent is located in the temple at Timna in the13th century B.C.E. [18] In

[9] 2 Kings 20:7.
[10] Mechilta D'Rabbi Ismael, p. 156.
[11] Omar, pp. 14-15.
[12] Auld & Steiner, pp. 74-75.
[13] This term was generally interpreted to refer to a tribe of giants that became extinct, see, for example, Dt. 2:11, 20;3:11.
[14] Jos. 15:8, 18:16.
[15] Parmentier, pp. 76-79. This scholar tries to associate Emek Rephaim with the area known as Bethesda where magical healing activity took place during the Roman period.
[16] Nu. 21:6-8.
[17] 2 Kings 18:4, cf. M. Pesahim 4, 10. The Torah forbids the use of "נחוש" (divination) (Lev. 19:26; Dt. 18:10) and it is no coincidence that in Hebrew the root of this word is identical to the root word 'נחש' meaning 'snake'. Jeffers brings a discussion on this subject, pp. 74-75 and reaches different conclusions.
[18] Stern, Encyclopedia, p. 1493.

later ages we recognize the serpent as the symbol of Askelpius, the mythological god of medicine. In any case we see that the Biblical approach is to reject any emblem that might have been used to recall miracle stories of the sick who had been cured in the Temple as was accepted practice in all the pagan temples of that period.

The conditions of hygiene and disease that prevailed in Jerusalem in the Biblical period may also be learned from the archaeological findings. In the City of David several toilet seats were found in private homes from the sixth century B.C.E.. These toilets were situated in small rooms, and each one had a square stone latrine, with a hole in the center. [Fig. 2] The toilet seats were located over cesspools.[19] These were private latrines which belonged to a well-to-do population of the upper classes which attest to the urban design and a highly developed awareness of sanitation. A study conducted on residues found in the cesspools at the City of David showed that they contained much ash which apparently was used to dry the waste material and to control the smell. In a study of fecal deposits, whipworm eggs and other parasites were recovered which exist in the digestive system. The scholars speculate that this may be related to the practice of irrigating the fields with water containing waste materials. [20]

Additional information about common diseases can be garnered from Paleopathological research. In burial caves that date to the end of the First Temple period (end of the 8th century-7th century BCE) on the western slope of Mt. Zion, the structure of the interred bones show signs that point to the fact that some of those interred were members of the same family and that the place served as a family burial plot. An examination of the teeth revealed that those interred in the cave, as opposed to most of the population in the Roman world, did not suffer from dental caries. 60% of the children showed changes in the eye sockets which indicate some form of disease characterized by anemia.[21]

Alongside of medicine, there is also information about the practice and profession of pharmacy in Jerusalem. The description of the burial of King Asa "sweet odors and divers kinds of spices prepared by the perfumer's[22] art" (Chron. II, 16:14) attests to the use of various spices which were compounded by professional pharmacists. Proficient particularly in that art were "some of the sons of the priests who made the ointment of the spices".[23] These priests were engaged in the preparation of the incense burned in the Temple, which according to the Bible had to be made from "a confection after the art of the perfumer". (Ex. 30:35) It appears that there was some connection between the practice of perfumery-pharmacy and of

[19] Chapman, pp. 4-8.
[20] Reinhard & Warnock, pp. 20-23.
[21] Davis & Cloner, pp. 16-19.
[22] The term used in the Koren translation for 'רוקחים' is 'perfumers' but must refer also to their function as 'pharmacists'.
[23] 2 Ch. 9:30.

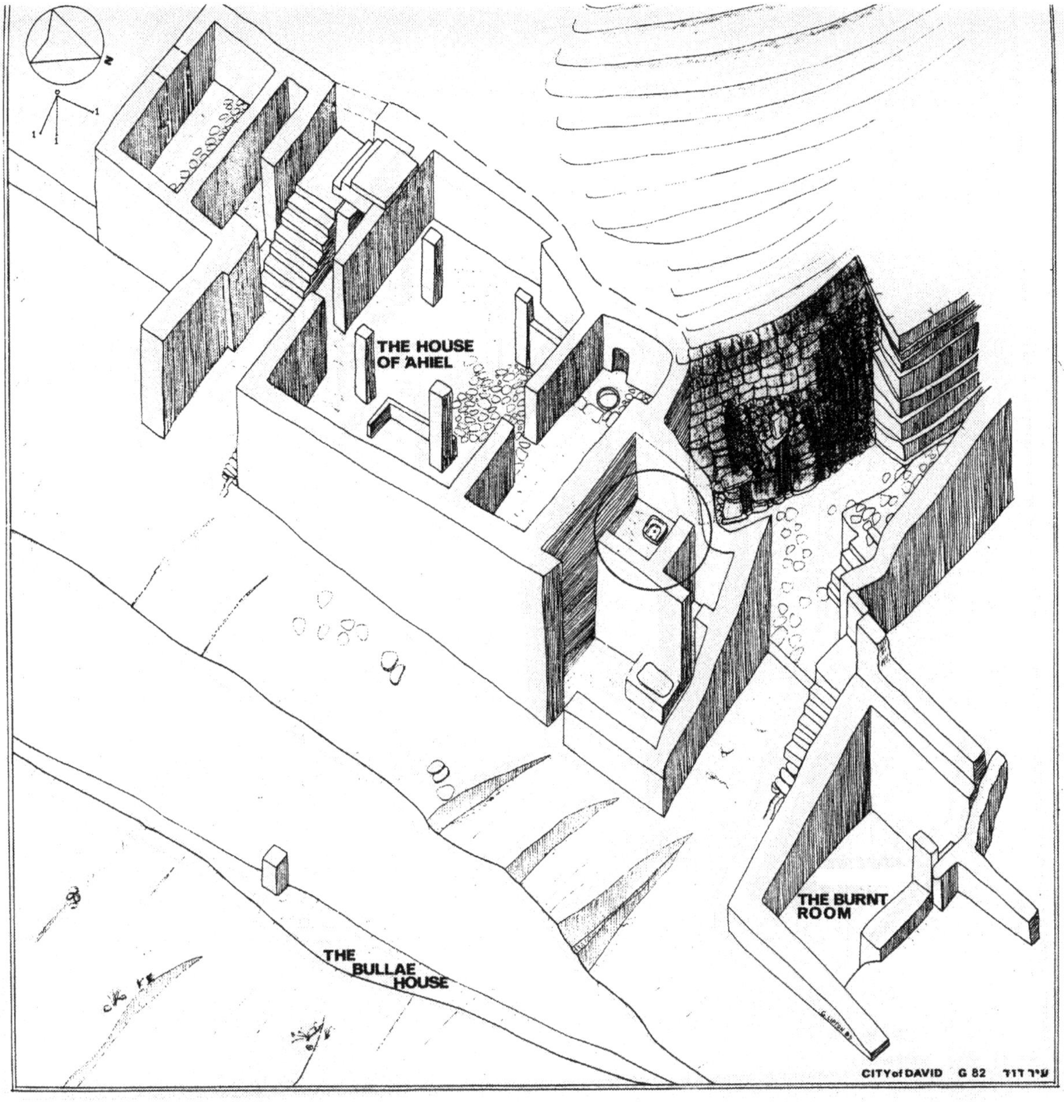

Figure 2: Latrine in Area E-3, City of David (Late Israelite Period [Iron Age])

medicine. The spices used in the incense were also used for medical purposes in ancient times[24] and preparing them employed the same technological methods. Furthermore, there are those who point to the burning of the incense as an act of health-enhancement. Thus, for example, Neufeld's article on hygiene conditions in ancient Israel, notes that incense when burned dispelled evil odors, exterminated pests, and served as an ecological disinfectant against sickness and plague. [25] An exposition of this theory may be found in the approach of Maimonides, the pre-eminent Jewish physician in the Middle Ages.[26]

[24] See: Crown, pp. 33-34; Ulman, pp. 194-205.
[25] Neufeld, pp. 427-432.
[26] Maimonides, Guide to the Perplexed, III, 45.

The Bible also mentions special "appointees" who were responsible for "the frankincense and the spices" [27], and they presumably sat in a special chamber.[28] These appointees were apparently associated in some kind of professional guild, generally within a limited family framework. In the list of those who built the walls of Jerusalem in the time of Nehemiah there is mention of Hananya son of the perfumers"[29], and it might be that this family attribution indicates that the profession was passed down from father to son.[30] There are those who think that one should not interpret the Hebrew word 'ben' in the text as 'son of' in the usual literal meaning of the word but rather as a member of the guild of perfumers. According to this reading, in the Biblical period the guild of perfumers, spice-growers, and perhaps even physicians represented a closed socio-economic class which protected its professional secrets.[31]

---

[27] 2 Ch. I 9:29.
[28] Neh. 13: 5,
[29] Neh. 3:8.
[30] Brin, pp. 85-86.
[31] Mendelsohn, pp. 17-21.

Chapter Two
Some facts about medicine in Jerusalem during the Roman Period

There is some information available on the subject of medicine in Jerusalem beginning in the first century BCE until the end of the second century CE, though the total amount of information is slight and cannot provide a clear and complete picture of the state of medicine in Jerusalem. Among the extant sources from the end of the Second Commonwealth are the Gospels and Josephus who mentions various aspects of medicine in his essays.[1] Most of the information from the Roman Period was derived from the Jewish sources: the Mishna, Tosephta, and rabbinical homilies [midrashim]. These sources do not belong to the body of medical literature, and the information they contain is random and incidental to a treatment of issues which are inarguably matters of Jewish law (*halacha*), such as: the laws of purity and impurity, the laws of the Passover sacrifice, and the Temple service.[2] The written sources are reinforced by the archaeological finds excavated in Jerusalem.

Sanitation and hygiene

Before reviewing the sources it should be stated that most were written during the period of Roman rule, and they undoubtedly reflect the Roman influence on the status of medicine throughout their empire. The Romans, continuing the Hellenistic rule which preceded them, promoted the science of medicine, particularly in the field of administration and in establishing well-developed sanitation facilities: the sewage system, bathhouses, toilets, sophisticated waterworks, and ecological legislation to preserve the public health. These activities were carried out with an eye to disseminating the Roman tradition and methods to all the provinces under their rule with an administrator's commitment to providing elementary services to its subjects.[3]

However, first and foremost the Romans ensured their own needs, particularly for their army with its numerous soldiers. Among the conspicuous examples of such projects in Jerusalem, we may mention the aqueducts which conveyed water from a distance of 20 km. south of Jerusalem to the city, thus making possible a regular supply of water to the city's population. The upper aqueducts showed inscriptions of the seventeen names of the centurions of the tenth Roman Legion dated to the second century CE. [4] Some of these aqueducts supplied water to the bathhouses used by the Roman army.[5] There were bathhouses in many

[1] See especially the work by Kottek who also cites many examples of Biblical stories which refer to various medical topics. These stories are described and interpreted in Josephus, according to the Roman realia as he knew it in his times.
[2] Dvorjetski, Health, pp. 7-31.
[3] Tasfrir, Eretz Israel, p. 40.
[4] Vetrali, pp. 149-161; Mazar, Survey, pp. 181, 189.
[5] Gichon & Isaac, pp. 117-123, no. 29.

of the military camps of the Roman legion in the Orient[6] which served as favored, popular places of recreation.[7] These bathhouses were built out of medical considerations as well, as part of the culture of the body, spirit, and personal hygiene, the product of the Hippocratic school of thought which attributed the greatest importance to preventive medicine.[8]

Josephus brings historical evidence referring to this practice in the Jerusalem region. Herod, on his way to Jerusalem after waging battle at the Canne River, went to wash himself "like any common soldier" [9]. According to him, Herod built bathhouses in Jerusalem at the tower of Phasael[10] and at the fortress of Antonia overlooking the Temple mount from the northwest.[11] A spacious bathhouse for the tenth Roman Legion was found in the southwestern section of the Temple Mount;[12] another bathhouse in Jerusalem whose construction is attributed to the soldiers of the tenth legion was found at Ramat Rachel[13] and Ein Yael.[14] Besides the bathhouses built for the army, in most of the residential homes of the favored Jewish elite, pools for bathing were found, alongside of ritual baths. These were not definitively Roman-style bathhouses but did include hypocaust systems designed for heating.[15]

Alongside the bathhouses, Jerusalem of the Roman Period also had public toilets (latrina) which were built for health reasons. A toilet from the Roman Period was found in the excavations southwest of the Temple Mount.[16] The written sources refer to a public bathroom that existed within the Temple site in Jerusalem: "A latrine of distinction and this was its distinction: when it was found to be locked, then they knew someone was inside; when found open, they knew that no one was inside."[17] It is very probable that this toilet was attached to the central drainage system of the Temple, which drained the blood and ashes from the outer altar to the aqueduct in the Temple Court, and from there the waste was conveyed to the Kidron River.[18]

Apropos a description of the walls of Jerusalem, Josephus mentions "Bethso" which was close to the Gate of the Essenes.[19] Yehosef Schwartz, upheld by most of the scholars after him, had proposed that this referred to a "beit tsoa" (privy) or a public toilet.[20] Yadin connected Beit Tsoa to the Gate of the Essenes and suggested that the location of this toilet was on the western side of the city, outside of the western city wall. He

---

[6] Stiebel, pp. 74-75.
[7] Davies, p. 66.
[8] Mazor & Bar-Natan, pp. 59-72.
[9] Josephus, JW, I 340.
[10] Josephus, JW, V 168.
[11] Josephus, JW, V 241.
[12] Mazar, Camp, p. 56.
[13] Aharoni, pp. 24-27.
[14] Edelstein, Villa, pp. 114-119.
[15] Avigad, pp. 142-143.
[16] Reich & Billig, pp. 38, 41.
[17] M. Tamid, I,1.
[18] M. Yuma, V, 6; Middot III,2; Har-El, pp. 310-313.
[19] Josephus, JW, V, 145.
[20] J. Schwartz, Grains, p. 335.

proposed that this public toilet served the Essenes living in that quarter. This facility was built as part of the strict laws of the Essenes which dictated that the privy must be located outside of the city as written in the Temple Scroll: "And you shall make for them a place outside of the city where they may go out there to the northwest of the city; houses with springs and pits within where the excrement may go down through them, so that it will not be visible to all, three thousand ells away from the city".[21] Other scholars believe that the Gate of the Essenes as well as the public privy were located in southeastern Jerusalem, in the lower section of the upper city, at the edge of the Tyropoeon Valley. This may have been one of the public toilets that served the residents of the capital and the pilgrims who came to spend the festivals.[22]

Purity and impurity

During the Second Commonwealth and even after the destruction of the Second Temple, there was a practice among the Jewish population (which was not restricted to peripheral sects like the Essenes) to strictly observe matters of ritual purity and impurity, not only within the confines of Jerusalem but throughout the country. This was also reflected in the local material culture as attested by the proliferation of ritual baths and various stone vessels found in the Jerusalem region.[23] While the stringent observance of the laws of purity - including bathing and immersion in water and avoiding contact with the dead - was carried out for strictly halachic motives, these practices did conform suitably with the facilities of hygiene and public health that were built at that same time under the influence of the Roman rule. Within this setting the rabbis of Jerusalem established several laws that were designed to guarantee the purity of the city to the pilgrims who stayed there[24], thereby also making a considerable contribution to the sanitation of the city and the health of its inhabitants. Among these regulations were a prohibition against accumulating refuse and dumping it within the city limits as well as a prohibition against raising animals and burying the dead within city limits.[25]

Professions Related to Medicine

A. Physicians

During the Roman Period the rabbinical sages enacted a regulation defining which institutions were required by a city, and this included listing both the facilities as well as the functionaries connected with public health:

[21] Yadin, Scroll, pp. 175-178.
[22] Har-El, p. 311.
[23] According to Jewish law, stone vessels are not subject to ritual impurity and during the Second Temple period, a stone vessel industry developed, centered around Jerusalem, see: Rimon, pp. 7-27.
[24] Safrai, Pilgrimage, pp. 135-136.
[25] T. Nega'im 6,a-b; Avoth de-Rabbi Nathan, vers. a, 35 (Schechter Ed.), p. 104); also vers. B, \39 (Shechter ed., pp. 107-108). For an extended discussion on this subject, see: Dvorjetski, Health, pp. 8-9.

"A Torah scholar is not permitted to live in a city which does not have these ten things … a bathhouse and public privy, a physician and a blood-letter"…[26]

It would seem that with these regulations the rabbinical sages wished to set forth elementary standards for a civilized society, apparently under the influence of the accepted standards of Roman society which reflected the modernization of their age. As we have noted, Jerusalem had bathhouses and public toilets but it also had the functionaries related to the medical profession.[27] The Jewish sources from the Roman Period refer to physicians who were active in the Jerusalem region. One may not rule out the possibility that this refers to people who specialized in the art of medicine according to the Greco-Roman school and served in the private sector. The distinguished physicians belonged to the elite of society. One of them may have been Tobias the Physician mentioned in the Mishna.[28] We have no additional information about this person other than his name and in the context of the text, it seems that he lived in Jerusalem itself or nearby. A later Talmudic source recounts that during the siege of Jerusalem in the year 69 CE, R. Johanan ben Zakkai asked the Roman emperor to send a physician to treat R. Zadok.[29] While that story seems to possess a mythic dimension, it also seems to contain a kernel of reality. There are scholars who wished to deduce from this that there were military doctors who served in the Roman army in Jerusalem.[30]

Additional evidence of the existence of a physician in Jerusalem may rest in an archeological finding. A sarcophagus found at Abu-Tor revealed the inscription "תרפט הנשבה"(=the captive physician). [Fig. 3] According to Rahmani the word 'תרפט' (tarafat) is derived from the Greek and has several meanings. He endorsed the possibility that this was the word for healer or physician.[31]

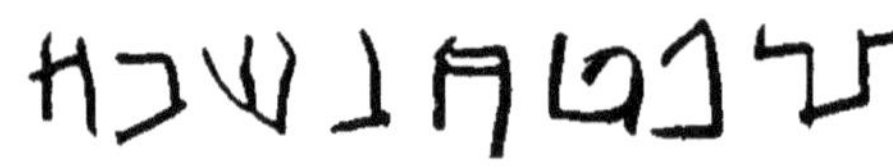

Figure 3: Inscription 'תרפט הנשבה" (=the captive physician?)

The term 'rofe' (=physician) also includes the concept of surgeon and these functionaries served the entire population of Jerusalem. The Mishna cites a tradition from the end of the Second Temple period regarding lepers who feared that their effected limbs would drop off and contaminate the Passover sacrifice. They would therefore visit a physician on the eve of Passover who would cut the afflicted limb in such a way so that it would not contaminate either the physician or the patient.[32]

---

[26] B. Sahnedrin, 17,b; J. Keddushin, 66d.
[27] The Roman city maintained urban physicians who received a salary for providing medical services to the city's population, see: Jones, p. 219.
[28] M. Rosh Hashana, I, 7.
[29] B. Gittin, 56b.
[30] Preuss, pp. 15, 441; Kottek, pp. 23, 193.
[31] Rahmani, pp. 96-97.
[32] M. K'ritot, III, 8.

B. Pharmacists

In addition to the physicians, there were pharmacists in Jerusalem during the Second Temple Period. It is natural that the Jewish halachic sources refer to this fact only from the religious perspective. The Mishna refers to the house of the family of "Avtinas" who were in charge of preparing the incense used in the Temple.[33] The incense was composed of eleven aromatic spices[34] and its preparation was considered a professional secret. According to a later tradition, the Avtinas family members had a "scroll of spices" [35], or in other words, they possessed professional literature on the subject. That same source indicates that they were also actively involved in gathering the spices for the incense as well as compounding them. The profession of gathering spices was also known during the Greek period as Rhizotomi and in Roman – Herbarii. This was a profession unto itself with a well-organized body of scholarship requiring knowledge in gathering and preserving herbs at the appropriate times and places.[36]

In the excavations at the upper city of Jerusalem (today, in the Jewish Quarter) a workshop from the end of the Second Temple Period was discovered with iron pestles, stone weights of various sizes, many different clay vessels, and perfume dishes made of glass. One of the weights bears the inscription "Bar Cataros", i.e., a son of the family of priest which is related to the 'cataros' (incense) which is known in the sources.[37] Avigad raised the theory that 'bar cataros' was engaged in the production of pharmaceutical products and perfumes that were supplied to the Temple, among others.[38]

C. Specialists

Among the functionaries at the Temple there was also mention of one Ben Ahiya who was responsible for those with "intestinal sickness".[39] This is an example of a specific medical specialist rather than a distinguished physician [40] who was supposed to supply medical services to all the sick who visited the Temple. At any rate this was not a person who practiced medicine through the use of magic. Intestinal disorders must have been the result of eating meat in the Temple courtyard where it may have spoiled, in the absence of proper refrigeration and preservation systems. In addition, the Talmud explains that the priests in the Temple would walk barefoot on the cold stone floor which caused them to catch a cold. Since the staple of their diet consisted of meat and wine which are hard to digest, this led to the priests' frequently falling

---

[33] M. Sh'ekalim IV,5.
[34] B. K'ritot, 6a.
[35] J. Sh'ekalim, 48d-49a.
[36] See, e.g., Theophrastus, IX, 8,5; Dioscorides, preface, p. 3.
[37] B. Pessahim, 57a; T. Menahot, 13, 21.
[38].Avigad, pp. 127-131
[39] M. Sh'ekalim, IV,5
[40] Preuss, p. 14.

sick with intestinal disorders. Ben Ahiya was a specialist in treating these symptoms by the use of wine mixed with certain medicinal drugs.[41]

Medicine in the Temples

Every temple was credited with events of a miraculous nature which represented a central element in the mind of the believers. Around the pagan temples revolved tales of the sick who were cured, barren women who became pregnant, etc. The religious establishment (particularly the priests) encouraged stories which enhanced the prestige of their temple and also naturally attracted believers and contributions. In light of this, Safrai noted that the paucity of stories about the sick who were cured in the Temple stands out as an exception.[42] Even the few sources which do point this out are problematic and do not reflect a familiarity with the reality of the Temple period or the central approach of the rabbinical sages. Thus, for example, one later midrash recounts: "And whoever was afflicted (outside of Jerusalem), as soon as he looked at the walls of Jerusalem, he would be cured."[43] This statement has no parallel and was stated in a rather low key without the further embellishment of any actual miracles which demonstrated the fulfillment of this promise. Another source tells of a religious ceremony that included encircling the Temple Mount, while reciting prayers:

> "And those who encircle from the left side are those who are in mourning and excommunicated and whoever has someone sick or has lost something...whoever has someone sick is told that He who dwells in this House will have mercy upon him. And if the sick person was capable of surviving, He would immediately have mercy upon him. And the story is told of a woman who fell sick and her daughter went up [to the Temple Mount] and encircled it and did not move from that place until they came and told her that she had been cured".[44]

The attitude described in this source is exceptional. This story appears in additional parallel versions but without alluding to any request for healing. It would seem that this source reflects the feelings of the public which tended to attribute to the Temple the hallmarks of a holy site such as those attributed to all the temples of that period.[45] In contrast, the sources which represent the official Jewish religious approach tried to play down the miraculous element in the Temple. An example of this may be seen in the difference between the version brought in the Tosephta and that brought by the compilers of the Mishna. The Tosephta relates: "There was a story about the mother of Rimatita (or Yarmita) whose daughter was sick, and she said, If my daughter recovers from her illness, I will donate her weight in gold. The daughter recovered and her mother

[41] J. Sh'ekalim, 48d.
[42] Safrai, Sanctity, p. 8.
[43] Avoth de-Rabbi Nathan, 35 (Shechter ed., p. 194); vers. B, 39 (p. 105).
[44] Treatise Semahot, VI, pp. 133-134.
[45] Safrai, Sanctity, p. 11.

went to Jersalam (Jerusalem) and gave her weight in gold". [46] While in this case the sick person was not actually cured in the Temple, this made it possible to convey the impression that dedicating money to the Temple may help in effecting a cure. However, in the parallel version that appears in the Mishna, there is no mention at all of any donation brought to the Temple in consequence of the daughter's recovery.[47] It thus emerges from the Mishna that the Mishnaic source wished to minimize mention of any activity in the Temple which might could be construed as having a magical curative effect. The object was to present a paradigm of a temple possessing a character different than that which was accepted in the pagan temples of that age. In following we will discuss two of the popular sacred healing sites in Jerusalem, located close to pools of water: the Pool of Bethesda and the Siloam. The historical sources and the archaeological finding show that during the Hellenistic period, pagan rituals were held there and with the spread of Christianity these sites continued to function as healing sites sacred to Christianity.

In the area around the Church of St. Anne near the Lion's Gate, there is a pair of large blessings identified as "the blessing of Beit Hisda". [Fig. 4] There are those who believe that the Greek and Latin name 'Bethesda' (John 5:2-9) is derived from the Hebrew name 'Beit Ashera' and not 'Beit Hisda'.[48] According to this suggestion, this referred to a site with a clear ritual significance which may have been rooted in a popular local, earlier ritual. Some archaeological excavations were held on the site which made it possible to reconstruct the dimensions and layout of the pools. According to the archeologists digging there, the pools had been excavated already back in the days of the Hasmonean dynasty (in an area that was then north of the walls of Jerusalem), in the second century BCE, but most of the findings are from the Roman Period. The remains include walls with sections of colored plaster, segments of mosaic, and a sophisticated system of waterways. According to the researchers, the finding is connected with a sanctuary of healing, that is, a complex of sacred waterworks used as a bath for curing the sick which was related to the cult of medicine of Askelpius. The relics found at the site, among them of vow offerings, attest to the rituals held there, as do the mementos left behind by the people who visited the site. Among the conspicuous findings are a broken relief in the facade of a building, and alongside it a snake with a figure making an offering of sheaves of wheat. The snake was one of the symbols of the cult of Askelpius. Likewise, a shard of marble identified as a foot was found bearing a Greek inscription noting the volunteer's name: Pompia Lukilia sacrificed (this foot)".[49] The use of a model of a hand or foot made of stone as a medical amulet was common in pagan ritual[50] and

[46] T. Arachin, 3, 1 (p. 545).
[47] M. Arachin, V, 1.
[48] Schik et al, 1888, 134. For other interpretations, see Parmentier, p. 79-81
[49] Benoit, pp. 48-57; Mauss, 1888; Ovadiah & de Silva 1984, pp. 223-234; Vincent & Abel 1926, pp. 694-695; Parmentier, pp. 75-76.
[50] Gersht, pp. 11-12.

the concept it reflected is expressed in the rabbinical literature of that period: "If a person finds a model of a hand or a foot, it is forbidden because such were used in idol worship".[51]

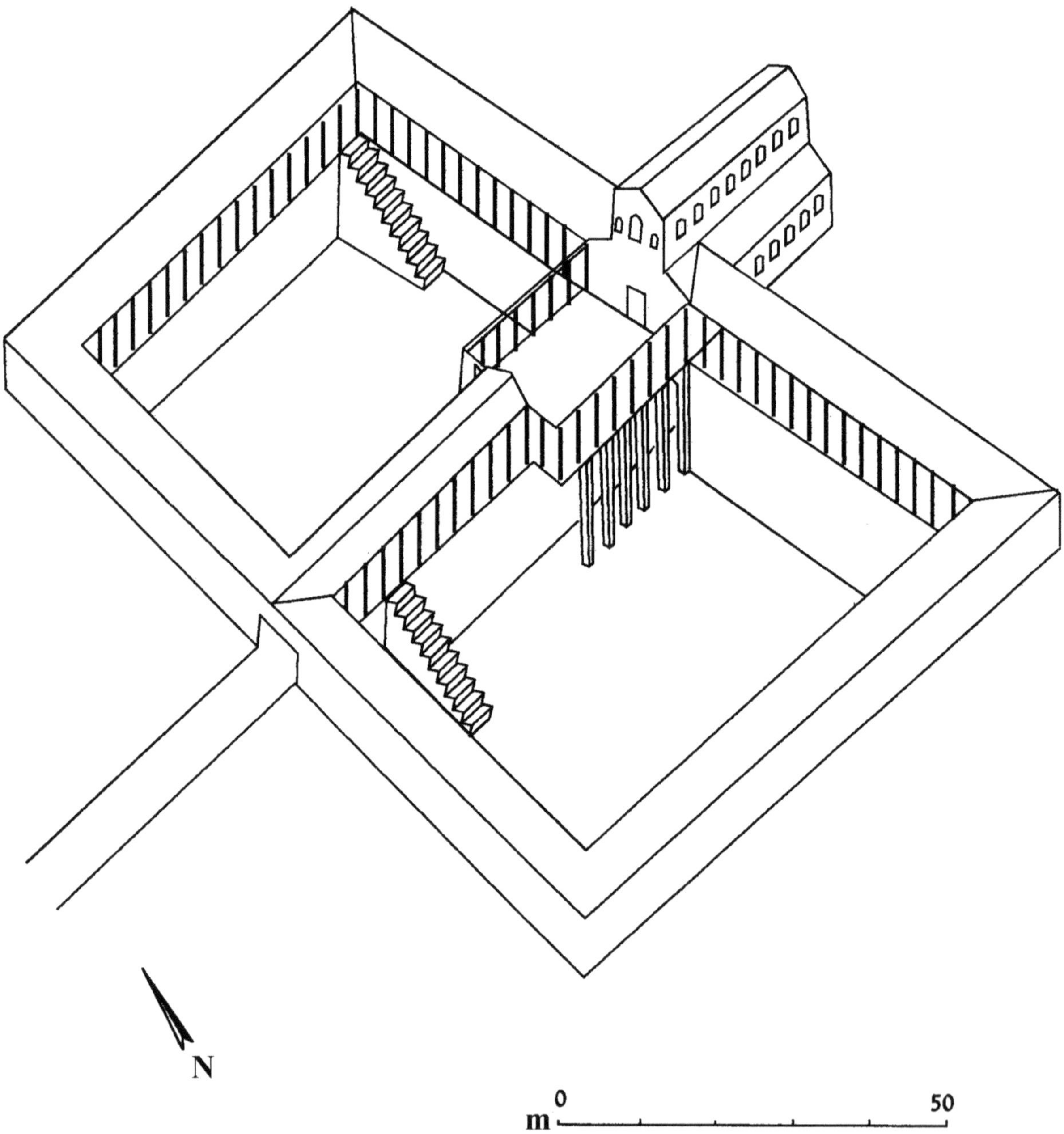

Figure 4: Pools of Bethesda (Byzantine Period)

[51] M. Avoda Zara, III, 2.

The blessing of Beit Hisda is mentioned in the New Testament as the site of healing where Jesus cured a sick person by miraculous means:

> "Now there is at Jerusalem, by the sheep gate, a pool which is called in the Hebrew tongue 'Bethesda' having five porches. In these lay a great multitude of impotent folk, of blind, lame, paralyzed, waiting for the moving of the water. For an angel went down at a certain season into the pool, and troubled the water; whosoever then first after the troubling of the water, stepped in was made well of whatever disease he had. And a certain man was there who had an infirmity thirty and eight years. When Jesus saw him lying there, and knew that he had been thus now a long time, he saith unto him, Wilt thou be made well? The impotent man answered him, Sir, I have no man when the water is troubled, to put me into the pool; but while I am coming, another steppeth down before me. Jesus saith unto him, Rise, take up thy bed, and walk. And immediately the man was made well, and took up his bed, and walked."[52]

This description shows that at that site there had been a large complex of buildings which was designed to take in the many sick visitors. The target group was the incurably ill for whom conventional medicine offered no hope. Treatment was therefore miraculous and connected to water. This corresponds to the method of healing associated with the cult of Askelpius. Medical treatment at Askelpion was carried out by the oracles of Askelpius and bathing in the waters was one of its characteristic hallmarks. Therefore the temples of Askelpius were usually built near sources of water and waterworks, and included lodgings for the use of those who came to be cured.[53] While the source in the New Testament does not explicitly state the existence of a pagan ritual on the site, it is apparent from the very fact that Christian tradition attributes a miraculous cure to Jesus on this site. According to this tradition, Jesus did not use water to cure the sick man, nor did he require any propitious occasion as in the cult of Askelpius. With this act he established his superiority over the local pagan ritual. Historically speaking, it does not matter whether Jesus ever did indeed visit this site and perform a miracle there. For our purposes, what is important is the Christian tendency to adopt the earlier pagan tradition and to reshape it with symbols more befitting its spirit. It is possible that after the spread of Christianity the site continued to be used as a ritual healing site. As in many other cases, Christianity, which wished to abolish the pagan distinguishing features which were prevalent among the common elements of the population, did not achieve its goal and thus was forced to compromise and accept it under Christian guise. The functioning of this site appears in a written source by the pilgrim of Bordeaux (333 CE):

[52] John 5:2-9.
[53] Edelstein, Asclepius, pp. 139-180; Walton, p. 44.

> "In Jerusalem beside the Temple there are two large pools, one to the right and the other to the left, built by Solomon, and inside the city are the twin pools with five porches called Bethsaida. People who had been sick for many years used to be cured there. The water of these pools is turbid and its colour is scarlet."[54]

In the Byzantine Period a church was built on the site, and it is described in many sources.[55]

Another healing site of pagan character which became sanctified in Christian tradition is the Pool of Siloam, located at the edge of the Tyropoeon Valley. The Siloam area was considered a sacred site even in Biblical times. [56] During the time of the Mishna the waters of the Siloam spring were considered pure and people would take water from there for libations and for waters of ritual purification.[57] As in other places, we find in the waters of Siloam a connection between water as a purifying force and its therapeutic properties. [58] According to a later midrash, which contains embedded elements of an earlier period, the waters of Siloam were known for their medicinal properties and are among the ten miracles that were performed in the Temple. Of the priests it was told: "After they had eaten much meat from the sacrifices, they would drink the waters of the Siloam and it would be digested in their intestines as food is digested."[59] This source reflects the popular tradition, one that came into conflict with the view cited in the Talmud, that the cure of the priests was effected by professional healers who specialized in this field.[60]

Near the pool of Siloam a pagan ritual also took place and it was called "Gad Yavan (or Yon)".[61] From the name in Hebrew, 'Gad' which means 'luck' one may speculate that the site was used for a pagan ceremony to the Greco-Roman goddess of luck, Tichi-Fortuna. Greco-Roman gods associated with water, among them the cult of "Tichi", are mentioned in the Talmud.[62] According to Greek mythology, the Greek gods dwelt near sources of water. There they would hold festivals, and bathing in a pool of water was considered a remedy for health and medicinal purposes. The rabbinical sages refrained from explicitly mentioning the name of this kind of idol worship because of the biblical injunction "neither let it be heard out of thy mouth" (Ex. 23:13) so that only a name already mentioned in the Bible was permitted to be mentioned. Thus they called the Greek ritual by an anachronistic name with the same meaning: the cult of Gad (Isaiah 65:11), the god of Fortune and success which was a familiar in the Canaanite pantheon.[63] Furthermore, in many cities in the land of Israel during the Greco-Hellenistic period, the goddess Ticha replaced the Semite god – Gad.

---

[54] CCSL, 1965, p. 589; Limor, pp. 30-31.
[55] Wilkinson, 1977, pp. 66, 84.
[56] Amar, Metamorphosis, pp. 207-222.
[57] M. Sukka, IV, 9; Para III, 2; T. Ta'anit I, 8.
[58] Patai, p. 32.
[59] Avoth de-Rabbi Nathan (Shechter ed., vers. A, 35 (p. 105).
[60] J. Shekalim, 48d.
[61] M. Zavim, I,5 and there are many versions. For other interpretations of "Gad Yavan (Yon)", see: Amar, Metamorphosis, p. 214.
[62] J. Avoda Zara, III, 3, 44d; Liberman, pp. 248-249.
[63] B. Sanhedrin, 63,b.

Historical and numismatic sources show that during the Roman period two temples were active in Aelia-Capitolina which were dedicated to the goddess Ticha and other gods.[64]

According to the descriptions of the rabbinical sages, the cult of "Gad Yavan (or Yon)" was held very close to the Siloam Spring at a distance of "like from Gadyon to Siloam which is like two immersions and two sponges"[65]. R. Shimon Bar Yohai makes a more precise estimate of distance as approximately one hundred cubits, [66] i. e. a distance of some fifty meters. The term "from Gadyavan to Siloam" indicates that a person who wished to immerse himself in the Siloam Spring which is apparently "the Pool of Alhamara" had to first pass through "Gadyon". This refers to the source of the Gihon from the Siloam tunnel, in a pool known today as "the (new) Pool of Siloam".[67] The accepted dating of the ancient remnants of the new Pool of Siloam is in the Roman Period.[68] Around the four walls of the pool, rows of columns have been reconstructed which are dated to that period because they were extant at the beginning of the Byzantine Period, as noted by the pilgrim from Bordeaux .[69]

At the archaeological excavations coins depicting Hygieia, daughter of Asklepius, were also found of Aelia Capitolina which are dated to the middle of the third century CE. Hygieia, the goddess of health and hygiene appears sitting on a rock and feeding a snake (which is also the symbol of Asklepius, the god of medicine). [Fig. 5] According to Meshorer, the cult of Hygieia which was usually located near sources of water took place near the Pool of Siloam, the only source of flowing water in the Jerusalem region. His theory is also based on the fact that therapeutic properties had always been attributed to the Siloam Spring , as previously mentioned.[70]. And indeed it was this site, at the same place known as the pagan site of "Gad Yavan" or at a temple attributed to Hygieia, that the Christians identified as the place where Jesus miraculously opened the eyes of a blind man:

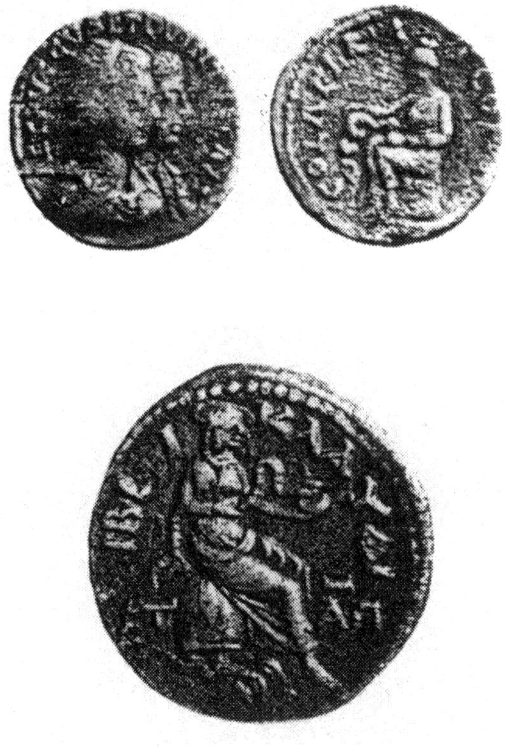

Figure 5: Coins of Aelia Capitolina depicting Hygieia, dated to the middle of the third century.

[64] Meshorer, Coinage, pp. 24-25, no. 39.
[65] T. Zavim, I, 5.
[66] T. Zavim, I, 1-11.
[67] Segal, p. 180.
[68] Bliss & Dickie, pp. 178-210.
[69] CCSL, 1965, p. 589; Limor, p. 30-31.
[70] Meshorer, Hygieia, pp. 17-18.

> "And as Jesus passed by, he saw a man who was blind from his birth... he spat on the ground and made clay of the spittle, and anointed the eyes of the blind man with the clay, and said unto him, Go, wash **in the pool of Siloam [which is by interpretation, Sent]**. He went his way, therefore, and washed, and came seeing."[71]

Here, too, we find the process by which Christianity re-fashions a pagan site in its own image. The functional properties and the target audience of the site are preserved while it is only the religious factor that changes. The site acquires renewed legitimacy firmly rooted in Christian scriptures, while the pagan ritual is delegitimized. According to the New Testament, there was a building at that time in Siloam which had collapsed and eighteen people were crushed to death underneath: "Or those eighteen, upon whom the tower in Siloam fell, and killed them, think ye that they were sinners above all men that dwelt in Jerusalem ?"[72] It may be that this referred to a building was connected with the cult of "Gad Yavan" or Hygieia, a ritual partaken of by the people who were killed on the site . In these words Jesus expressed implied criticism of all the people of Jerusalem who took part in pagan rituals.

The two miraculous cures attributed to Jesus[73], at Beit Hisda and at Siloam, are recounted only in the Gospel of John and the explanation for it is not the subject of our discussion here. However, it would be appropriate to comment on the New Testament as a source for learning about the history of medicine of that time. In the first three Gospels as well as in the book of Revelation, there are more references to medical subjects than in any other document from the Second Temple Period.[74] In all of them, the persona of Jesus is revealed as a messenger of God and a popular healer employing magic to effect his cures.[75] In one of the sources it is stated explicitly that Jesus declared of himself in Jerusalem that "Behold, I cast out demons and I do cures".[76]

It would seem that the manner is which Jesus was portrayed as a magical healer and the methods of healing used in the pagan temples in Jerusalem and the environs during the Hellenist-Roman Period may explain why over time the fundamental approach which crystallized in the sources of later Jewish law wished to downplay medical activity of a mystical nature in the Temple in Jerusalem. The various sources, Jewish, Christian, and other cults also reflect the different trends and ways of thinking that were prevalent during the Helleno-Roman period regarding the ideal method of healing and determining the legitimate status of the conventional physician and the possibility of a mortal physician intervening in acts

---

[71] John, 9: 1-11.
[72] Luke, 13:4.
[73] Kee, pp. 88-94.
[74] Amundsen & Ferngren, pp. 2934-2956.
[75] Hogan, pp. xiii-xiv.
[76] Luke, 13:32. On Jesus as a sorcerer, see the famous book by Smith which aroused many responses.

of Providence.[77] However, beyond that, the sources show that there was extensive and diversified medical activity in Jerusalem at that time.

[77] See, e.g., Amundsen & Ferngren, p. 2952.

Chapter Three
From Byzantine Rule to Muslim Rule

This chapter deals with the history of medicine in Jerusalem and the environs in the 6th to11th centuries. The chronological purvey of this work was in effect determined by the information available to the researchers, since significant information about materia medica and outstanding physicians in Jerusalem in particular and the land of Israel in general only begins to appear from the tenth century onward. The 300-year period of Islamic rule and all of the preceding periods are conspicuous for the paucity of material available. At the same time there is no lack of material relating to the nature and development of medical science in the Byzantine period as compared with the early Arab period.

Various studies show that the transitional period between the Byzantine and Arab period in the land of Israel must be seen more or less as of one uniform piece. The Arab conquest did not bring about any great upheaval, nor did the political revolution that was transpiring in the region lead to any immediate change in the civilization and its material and spiritual culture. In many cases there is even evidence of a continuation of the patterns of the Byzantine rule. This is true to a large extent for all matters relating to medicine and the nature of medicine in greater Jerusalem. This study demonstrates the continuity of the medical system during the Early Islamic Period (640-1099) as it had been shaped in the Byzantine Period. This continuity is reflected in the continued predominance of Christian doctors in the field of medicine both in the practice and teaching of medicine, in preparing 'theriac' (an anti-toxin serum), in operating the hospitals (general and leper hospitals) and consecrated healing institutions by the monks and clergymen, as well as in the provision by the Muslim regime of the funds for the medical infrastructure in a format similar to the type that had operated during the period of Byzantine rule.

In addition, it must be remembered that on the broader cultural level there was no conflict between the Muslims and the Christians in the Middle East in any of the matters relating to the branches of science. Already in the early Byzantine period, with the acceptance of the Galenic medical tradition by the Christians, Christianity became in effect the continuer of the classical medical culture. Later, following the Islamic conquests, it was chiefly the Christians who translated the writings of classical medicine into Arabic, and this constituted a cultural link connecting the east with the west as well as the ancient period with the Middle Ages.

Our study shows that the chronological division between the Byzantine and Muslim periods is often an artificial one; some of the information that appears as a description of the Byzantine period also applies to the Arab period, and vice-versa. Furthermore, the information on outstanding physicians and the use of materia medica, most of which only appears in the Arab period, undoubtedly reflects the reality during the

Byzantine period as well. At the same time, one cannot ignore the fact that there is a discrepancy between the two periods in the amount of available information, and the different fields of interest characteristic of each period constitute a difficult methodological problem requiring much prudence in interpreting the information.

The Byzantine Period (324-640)

Medicine during the Roman Period represents a continuation of the Greek medical tradition. The Romans advanced the science of medicine particularly in terms of bureaucratic organization, in establishing well-developed sanitation facilities: sewage systems, bath-houses, sophisticated water projects, and ecological legislation to preserve public health. The Romans developed the specialty of military medicine, which included army doctors and the establishment of military hospitals. The military needs of the Romans, their organizational and administrative talents, together with economic interests were important factors in shaping the institution known as the hospital. Hospitals served military personnel and a limited sector of the population which was connected to the ruling power.

While one may attribute the development of medical institutions to the Romans, the institutionalization and distribution of medical services must be credited to the Byzantines. At first Christianity rejected classical rational medicine because of its pagan hallmarks, but with the firmer establishment of Christianity, it adopted the principles of the Greek-Roman medical tradition.[1] As Christianity became an official religion, the Church took over the role of caring for the needs of the sick, transferring it from the responsibility of the civil government. The church undertook the goal of supplying social services to the entire local Christian population, to the church personnel, and to the pilgrims. Legislation by the Roman Empire granted the church the authority for enforcing social laws and funding the establishment of a well-developed infrastructure of public health.[2] In this way the church also managed to extend its influence over the local population and to reinforce its status as part of the ruling authority. The combination of the religious and governmental authorities within the Byzantine Empire had a decisive effect on the development and shaping of the system of medicine in the land of Israel during this period as well as after the Muslim conquest.

Medicine Within the Monastic Movement

Operating and deploying the medical system was carried out primarily by the monastic movement which had a strong influence on the Church, the government, and society as a whole. One of the major centers of monasticism was the Judean Desert which, on the one hand, was suitable for a life of solitude while at the

[1] Allan, pp. 450-451.
[2] Downey, pp. 199-208; Ashkenazi, Involvement, p. 46.

same time it was close to Jerusalem and the vigorous Christian activity taking place there. In that sense the description given by various Byzantine sources to the Judean Desert region is most fitting, as they labeled it "the desert of Jerusalem"[3] and the monks of the Judean Desert were known as "the monks of Jerusalem". In Jerusalem itself, especially on Mount Zion and the Mount of Olives, there were monastic centers which were more closely connected with the Christian pilgrim movement.[4] Some of the large monasteries in the Judean Desert also had hostels in Jerusalem, and through these organizations they maintained direct and uninterrupted contact with the life and visitors of the city.[5]

During the Byzantine Period, the institution of medicine developed, interestingly enough, in the east rather than in the west: in Asia Minor, Syria, and the land of Israel which were influenced by the extensive growth of the Christian population.[6] The origins of the institutionalization of Church-related medical services is attributed to Basil, founder of the Cappadocian monastic movement (middle of the fourth century). Basil taught his followers to take an active role in the life and needs of the community and to become involved in helping and caring for the sick even beyond the confines of their monastery.[7] This tradition had a powerful influence on the monks of the Judean Desert, most of whom had come from Asia Minor.[8] These monks were very involved in leadership roles in Jerusalem and in the care of the sick of the city.[9]

Among the monastic movements, one finds involvement in the practice of conventional medicine, but in addition, the art of healing is practiced based on miraculous religious elements.[10] One may read about the involvement of the monks of the Judean Desert from the writings of the monastic fathers. Thus for example, Theodosius (430-529) has been described as a physician full of compassion for the poor and the infirm sick, such as the blind and lame.[11] It is told of Euthymius that he healed several people miraculously.[12] He was especially well known among the local population when he cured the half-paralyzed son of the leader of the Saracens by means of prayer.[13] This fact takes on special importance inasmuch as Euthymius was one of the heads of the monastic movement in the Judean Desert in the fifth century, and he made a prominent contribution to the shaping of monastic life and the dissemination of Christian teachings among the nomads.

From the time of Euthymius there is no shortage of accounts of cures characterized by religious symbolism in the Jerusalem region, particularly in those cases where conventional medicine had failed to produce a

---

[3] Hirschfeld, Monasteries, p. 13.
[4] Gayger, p. 231.
[5] Hirschfeld, p. 184.
[6] Miller, Birth, pp. 68-71; Allan, p. 446.
[7] Miller, Birth, pp. 118-120; Allan, pp. 448-449; Ashkenazi, Curing, pp. 34-36; Ashkenazi, Involvement, p. 45.
[8] Hisrchfeld, Monasteries, pp. 94-95.
[9] Price, pp. 26-29 in the preface; Patrich, Monasticism, pp. 149-151.
[10] Ashkenazi, Involvement, pp. 44-45.
[11] Theodosius, pp. 34-35.
[12] I.e., the curing of madness in a young boy from the village of Aristobolias; Schwartz, pp. 22-23.
[13] Schwartz, pp. 18-21.

satisfactory solution. One of the common forms of healing involved the use of oil consecrated from relics.[14] This phenomenon is also known in other parts of Israel.[15] Consecrated oil from the grave of Euthymius was used to cure peasants from the Jerusalem region and sick aristocrats who visited the city.[16] It is also told of Sabas, the disciple of Euthymius, that he cured a man from Medaba by anointing him with oil from the holy cross, after he was wounded on the Mt. of Olives and the conventional healer did not succeed in healing him.[17] Sabas was also asked by the Patriarch of Jerusalem to come to treat his sister who fell victim to severe pains. He succeeded in curing her after she had despaired of the physicians.[18] A similar account is brought in relation to a nun by the name of Melania who sojourned in Jerusalem in the fifth century. The nun was brought a young woman whose mouth had been sealed shut by a demon which took possession of her, and consequently it was feared that she would die of hunger. All of the efforts of the physicians who concocted various remedies were to no avail. The author of the chronicle relates that when the art of medicine was found ineffective, the girl was brought to Melania who cured her with oil consecrated from holy relics.[19] It is told of Cyriacus, one of the leading monks, that during his sojourn in the Natoupha Desert, he succeeded in curing a youth afflicted with epilepsy using prayer and oil from the holy cross.[20]

As these examples demonstrate, the chronicles written by the leaders of the monastic movement either tell little of outstanding physicians and conventional methods of healing or else they belittle them. These sources naturally tend to highlight the miraculous and religious in medical treatment which to their view was more effective than conventional medicine. However, from what is not told, we learn of the existence of outstanding physicians who were engaged in medical practice in the Jerusalem region. One must furthermore be careful to avoid the mistaken impression that the monastic movement rejected conventional medicine. Along with the miracle cures, monks played a prominent role in disseminating conventional medicine, and as part of this effort served outstanding physicians who gave treatment based on the medical tradition of their times.

Hospitals

During the Byzantine Period several hospitals were built in the Jerusalem region and the Judean Desert, which became part of a network of institutions devoted to charity, nursing, and hospitality, such as old age homes, soup kitchens, and hostels. These institutions have been extensively described by Ya'akov

[14] Price, pp. 33, 37.
[15] See: Dauphin, pp. 40-42.
[16] Schwartz, p. 68. See in particular the series of tales in chapters 52-55, pp. 76-77.
[17] Schwartz, p. 136.
[18] Schwartz, p. 170.
[19] Melanie, pp. 247-249.
[20] Subsequently he was also brought a patient who was afflicted with an evil spirit and he treated him in the same fashion. See: Schwartz, p. 228.

Ashkenazi.[21] In Byzantine sources, these institutions are referred to by different terms derived from the Greek: xenon (or xenodochium), nosokomeion, and later in Latin giving us the term 'hospital'.[22] Since it is not always clear whether the reference is to a true hospital or to institutions offering hospitality or nursing, we will relate in this study only to accounts that refer directly to care of the sick. One tells of a hospital in Jericho[23] at the "Great Laura" near Tekoá (Dir Mar Saba). Sabas established a hospital whose staff included a physician.[24] This hospital provided medical service to all the affiliated monasteries in the area.[25] At the monastery of Theodosius there apparently were three separate hospital buildings: one for monks within the confines of the monastery itself, another building for laymen (apparently for payment), and the third for the indigent. There was a separate medical staff in each of the hospitals who treated the sick according to instructions given by Theodosius and using medications that he concocted himself.[26]

Within the city of Jerusalem during the Byzantine Period there were at least two hospitals which could provide institutionalized medical services to a large population. These hospitals and other institutions of philanthropy were usually established close to churches and administered by the monks.[27] The first hospital apparently was built by Eudocia in the fifth century in the patriarchal quarter surrounding the Holy Sepulcher. This hospital is mentioned in an inscription from Gai Ben Hinnom: "The grave of Avgenius of the Hospital of the Patriarch". [28] This hospital gave medical treatment to the residents of greater Jerusalem and the monks of the region. It seems that this is the hospital referred to in the days of Euthymius (middle of the fifth century) who was active in the time of Eudocia. In this context the account is told of a monk who was brought by the residents of the village of Lazariun (al-Ázariya) close to Jerusalem to the hospital in the holy city. [29] There is also an account of a monk from the laura at Pharan (near Éin Pharrah) who was stricken in his abdomen and who was sent to the patriarchal hospital.[30]

In addition to the patriarchal hospital, another hospital was established in Jerusalem in the middle of the sixth century. This hospital was part of the church complex at the Church of the New Miriam "The Nea" which was built by Justinianus (ruled 527-565). According to Cyrilius, building a hospital "for the benefit of foreigners who take sick" was done at the request of Sabas,[31] one of the prominent monks in the land of Israel of the sixth century who was one of the disciples of Euthymius. At first this hospital had one hundred

[21] Ashkenazi, Curing, p. 35.
[22] On the various terms that describe charitable institutions and how they developed, see: Miller, Birth, pp. 21-27; Miller, Knights, pp. 710-711. Incidentally the Hebrew word for inn 'אכסניא, [akhsania] was borrowed from the Greek 'xenon'.
[23] Theodorus, p. 42. According to Ashkenazi, Curing, p. 41, there was also a hospital at the laura of Kelmon (near Éin Hajla) and this is based on the life of Ciriacus (Schwartz, p.226), However, from the text it would seem that this was apparently an inn rather than an institution of healing.
[24] Schwartz, pp. 117, 131.
[25] Patrich, Monasticism, p. 150.
[26] Theodosius, p. 41.
[27] Tsafrir, Zion, p. 14.
[28] Macalister, pp. 232-234.
[29] Schwartz, p. 70.
[30] Joannes Moschus, p. 2896.
[31] Schwartz, p. 175.

beds and later, this number doubled. The operation of the hospital was funded by the emperor Justinianus and was allocated 1850 solidi per annum.[32] Procopius notes that close to the church were two inns which offered lodging and medical treatment for the poor.[33] It would seem that this hospital was intended to offer a solution for the stream of pilgrims to the city at that time while the patriarchal hospital served the local population primarily. One may learn of the dimensions of the hospital associated with the Nea complex from the account given by the pilgrim from Piacenza who visited the city circa 570:

> "From Sion we went to the basilica of Saint Mary, with its great congregation of monks, and its great houses for men and women. In catering for travelers they have a vast number of tables, and more than three thousand beds for the sick."[34]

It appears that the number of beds mentioned by this source is exaggerated, but the general appraisal may certainly be accepted that the building contained a large number of beds. The beds, incidentally, were an item of furniture generally intended only for the sick, while the monks and guests at the monasteries and hostels used to sleep on pallets or mats spread on the floor.[35] From the description given by the Piacenza pilgrim, one may also learn of the role played by the monks and church officials in operating a medical institution that was primarily designed for pilgrims and of its involvement in the civil government, whose funding was essential in building and maintaining such a large medical system. The Nea Church inaugurated in 543 was destroyed in the Persian conquest (614). When we later discuss the source of the inspiration for the Hospitaller medical institution which housed hundreds of patients in the Crusader Period in Jerusalem, we may confidently point to the Nea hospital as the prototype of the public medical institutions which were known in the East.

Consecrated institutions of healing

As we have seen in Chapter Two, during the Helleno-Roman Period, at least two sites were known to have functioned as healing spas regarded as holy: the Pool of Siloam and the Pools of Bethesda (the Sheep Pool). Both were located near pools of water which certainly made them eligible to serve simultaneously as both healing spas and holy sites. These sites were considered therapeutic with a reputation for curing hopeless diseases, drawing their unique qualities from a divine power. Pagan rituals were carried out at these sites, and with the spread of Christianity, these sites continued to function as healing spas, gradually acquiring distinctly Christian features.[36]

[32] Schwartz, p. 177.
[33] Procopius, Buildings, V 6, 25.
[34] CCLS, p. 141; Wilkinson, p. 84.
[35] Hisrchfeld, Monasteries, p. 236.
[36] Amar, Metamorphosis, pp. 207-222; Benoit, pp. 48-57; Bliss & Dickie, pp. 178-210; Schick et al, pp. 111-134.

We have no evidence that the Pools of Bethesda continued functioning as a clearly-defined healing site in the Byzantine Period although therapeutic qualities were still ascribed to its waters by virtue of the Christian and popular traditions that were prevalent among the local population in later generations as well.[37] In contrast, the information about the Pool of Siloam is more solidly based. During the Byzantine period this site became institutionalized, with the Christian elements becoming more pronounced. Events connected with Jesus (John 9:1-11) and the site's therapeutic qualities were a lodestone not only for believers from the surrounding area but also for the many pilgrims who came there from afar. The development of this site must be seen against the background of the increased traffic of pilgrims in the land of Israel in general and against the background of the entire development of medical services that accompanied it.

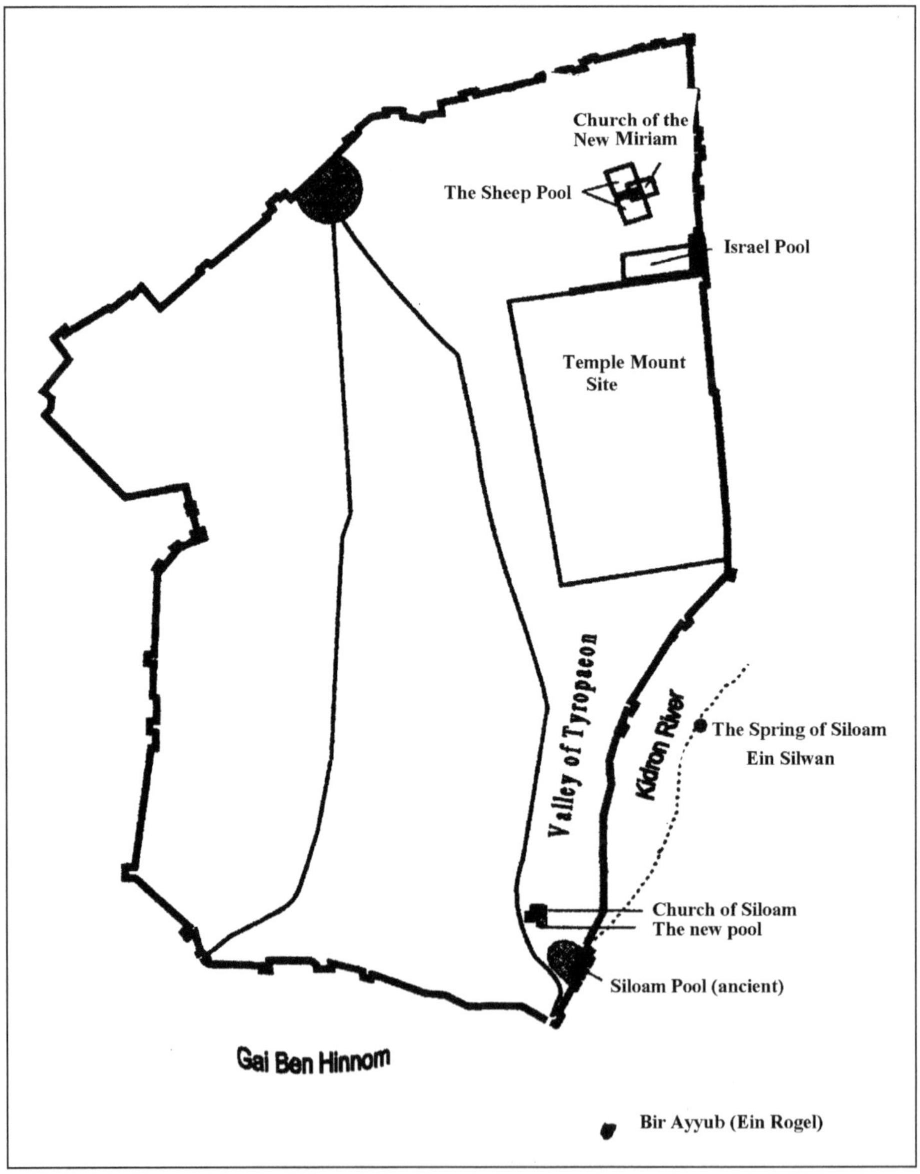

Figure 6: Sacred healing sites in Jerusalem, early Byzantine period: (pools of the sheep) and Siloam.

[37] Amar, Metamorphosis pp. 207-211.

The Siloam site was operated by monks who served at the site, and it was accorded support and recognition by the local Byzantine rule. The Empress Eudocia built the "Church of Siloam" above the site in the middle of the fifth century and an inn for guests which was designed to offer services to the many pilgrims and sick people who visited the site.[38] In the cemetery at Silwan an inscription was found with a reference to the hospital. Some scholars propose that it was on the Mount of Olives[39] but one may not rule out the possibility that this referred to a medical institution connected to the Church of Siloam. This was a religious institution with both a tourist as well as a medical disposition. We find evidence of this in the words of the Piacenza pilgrim who describes the miraculous cures at the site:

> "Siloam has two basins constructed of marble, which are separated from each other by a screen. Men wash in one and women in the other, to gain a blessing. In these waters many miracles take place, and lepers are cleansed." [40]

The remnants of the Siloam basins which have been uncovered and well-preserved attest to the functional planning; this consisted of the Byzantine entrance and the pool of Siloam which was integrated into this complex.[41] The description of the Pool of Siloam given by the Piacenza pilgrim recalls the description that he brings in another place in reference to Hammat Gader.[42] At Hammat Gader, too, Eudocia contributed generously to renovate the site[43] and in both cases the reference was to consecrated healing spas that continued to operate even after the Muslim conquest. At Hammat Gader there is clear evidence that the site was adopted by the Umayyad regime which in effect continued the arrangements of the previous government.[44] At Hammat Gader as at the Siloam in Jerusalem, one may observe the familiar model of a healing spa that bears a distinctly religious nature[45] which continues to operate over time under the various religious and governmental aegis. The sources of the Muslim period do not explicitly mention a church near Siloam but the site apparently continued to operate. The church which had been sacked during the period of the Persian conquest (614) was evidently reconstructed later.[46]

The map of Medaba dated to the sixth century or by a different proposal, to the second half of the seventh

[38] Holum, pp. 218-219; Ovadiah, Corpus, p. 91; Ashkenazi, Involvement, p.46.
[39] Germer-Duraud, p. 566; Milik, p. 149.
[40] CCLS, p. 142; Wilkinson, p. 84.
[41] Vincene & Abel, pp. 860-864; Bliss & Dickie, pp. 178-210.
[42] Following is his description: "...three miles from the city, there are hot springs called the baths of Elijah. Lepers are cleansed there, and have their meals from the inn there at public expense. The baths fill in the evening. In front of the basin is a large tank. When it is full, all the gates are closed, and they are sent in through a small door with lights and incense, and sit in the tank all night. They fall asleep, and the person who is going to be cured sees a vision." See: CCLS, p. 132; Wilkinson, p. 81; Hirschfeld, Hammat, pp. 5-6. The interlude in the water and the cure by a night vision strongly recalls the nature of the cure that was the practice at the Asclepius Temples.
[43] Green & Tsafrir, pp. 29-30.
[44] Green & Tsafrir, pp. 28-36; Hasson, pp. 97-101.
[45] Dvorjetski, Springs, p. 25.
[46] Bahat, Layout, p. 53, note 162.

century after the Arab conquest,[47] depicts many structures whose identification is disputed by scholars:

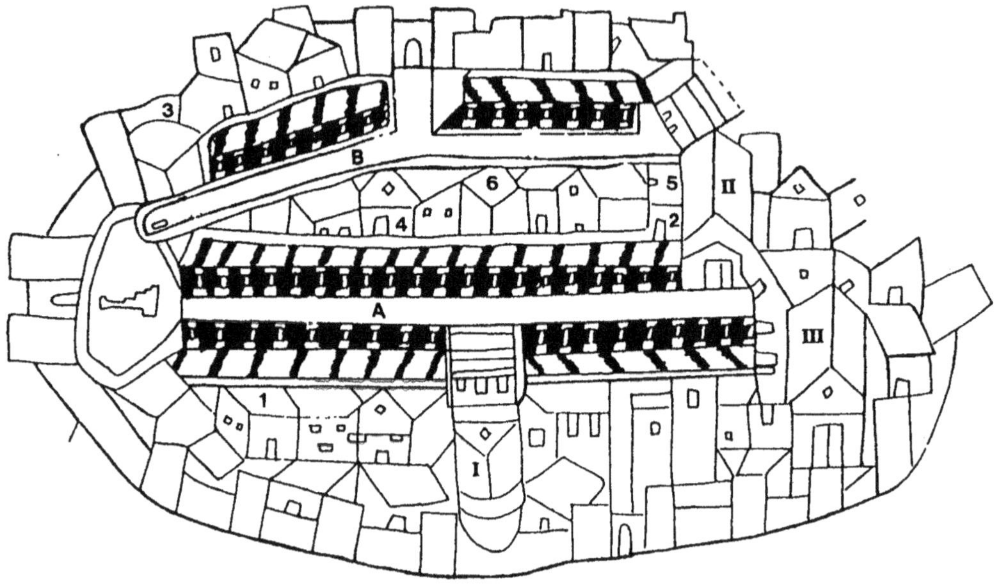

Figure 7: Medaba Map (sketch) of nursing and medical institutions in Jerusalem in the early seventh century (according to Ashkenazi)

Key:

1. Hospital of the Patriarch near the Church of the Holy Sepulcher
2. The Royal Hospital established by Emperor Justinianus
3. Institution for elderly women established by Johannan Euderinus of Byzantine near the Porbatica Church
4. Church of Cosmas and Damianos (in memory of two saints who were popular healers: ’αυάργυροι)
5. Hospitals for indigent pilgrims established by the Emperor Justinian (?)
6. The Royal Home for the Aged

I Church of the Holy Sepulcher
II The ‘Nea’ Church
III Church of Zion

A Cardo maximus
B Cardo decomanus

hospitals (of the Patriarch or the Nea), hostels and monasteries among others.[48] [Fig. 7]. Some scholars identify in one of the structures the basilica of the Church of Siloam. Above the basilica is a square structure with a domed roof.[49] If this is indeed the basilica structure above the Church of Siloam, then the overhead structure may have been used as an inn or hospital. The healing properties of the Pool of Siloam which was enclosed in the church are mentioned by Sophronius, patriarch of Jerusalem, in the beginning of the Islamic conquest.[50] We have additional evidence that the site continued to function only from a later period, in the description given by a Persian traveler, Nasir Khusraw, who visited Ain Silwan [the Spring of Siloam] in 1047:

[47] Bahat, Proposal, pp. 74-75.
[48] Tsafrir, Zion, pp. 308, 341-342.
[49] Tsafrir, Zion, p. 339.
[50] Wilkinson, p. 171.

> "It is said that when anyone washes from head to foot in this water he obtains relief from his pains, and will even recover from chronic maladies. There are at the spring many buildings for charitable purposes, richly endowed; and the Holy City itself possesses an excellent Bimaristan (or hospital) ... Great numbers of (sick) people are here served with potions and lotions; for there are physicians who receive a fixed stipend, and attend at the hospital."[51]

The term 'hospital' appears in the Persian source as 'Bimaristan'. This traveler does not state who were the people who come to visit the site or who operates and pays for it but the connection he draws between the description of Ain Silwan and the hospital of Jerusalem is not a chance one. From other sources we learn that in the First Muslim Period the medical profession in the land of Israel in general and the Jerusalem region in particular was largely controlled by Christians who were the dominant component among the local population. Furthermore, even among the Muslims, distinctly Christian beliefs and traditions prevailed which were current in the land of Israel during the Byzantine Period.[52] Consequently there was nothing to prevent the Muslim rule from officially recognizing this institution and it may even have supported it, although on a practical basis, the Siloam site was operated by Christian monks. The division of authority where the civil authority was responsible for building hospitals and the Church, for maintaining and operating them, had in fact been determined previously at the beginning of the Byzantine period.[53] As in many cases, here, too, we are witness to continuity and to the Muslim rule adopting the methods of the Byzantine rule in the Land of Israel.

Another explanation for the description given by Nasir Khusraw is that this was a conventional hospital, and then, two possibilities may be raised for identifying it.

The first possibility is that Nasir Khusraw is referring to the hospital of the Patriarch which had been established in the Byzantine Period; the second possibility is that this was yet another hospital which served all of the residents of the city. It should be noted that except for this account, there is no additional information about any hospital in Jerusalem throughout the entire First Muslim Period.[54] If indeed there were no special medical institutions for the Muslim community, then it is reasonable that it used the medical services provided by the Christians who were the only agency which could have provided public medical services. In such a reality, the central government would also have been compelled to recognize the Christian medical institution. However, even if we assume that that the reference is to a hospital built by the Muslim

---

[51] Khusraw, p. 21.
[52] Amar, Tradition, pp. 23-34.
[53] Ashkenazi, Involvement, p. 43.
[54] Some scholars think that among the charitable works established by Charlemagne in Jerusalem (ca. 800) was a hospital. However, sources indicate an inn that was designated for pilgrims and there is no clear-cut evidence that it was used for medical treatment. See the description by Bernard in Wilkinson, p. 142. According to Delaville (pp. 6-9) the buildings erected by Charlemagne continue the buildings built by Gregorius the Great in 603 which were destroyed apparently during the Persian conquest (614). On the building projects of Charlemagne and later, of the Amalfitans, see: Bahat, Layout, pp. 48-52.

regime, then it is highly probable that this was influenced by the Byzantine tradition.[55] Besides this, one must note that there were physicians who worked privately in Jerusalem during the First Muslim Period and this will be discussed later.

Leper Hospitals in Jerusalem

It is from the Piacenza pilgrim that we learn about the care of lepers in Jerusalem during the Byzantine Period (from 570). According to his account, the lepers would go to the pool of Siloam to seek a miracle cure from their affliction. [56] In the First Muslim Period the Church of Saint Stephen which stood outside the city wall was rebuilt in Jerusalem. The church also housed a leprosarium which, according to the commemoratorium circa 808, accommodated fifteen lepers and two clergymen.[57]

In the Judean Desert, monks established hospitals for lepers, since treating and coming into contact with them was forbidden within the city limits of Jerusalem. According to a fourteenth century historian, Eudocia (d. 460) built a hospital, apparently near Herodian, for four hundred patients who were "afflicted with the holy disease".[58] The monastery of Theodosius (est. 476) apparently also specialized in treating leprosy patients.[59] In addition to the written sources there is pathological evidence of the presence of leper colonies in the monasteries of the Judean Desert which were close to Jerusalem. In two monasteries bone fragments were discovered of scores of people who had been afflicted with leprosy and tuberculosis; in the Martyrius Monastery and in the Monastery of John the Baptist (Katzar al-Yahud). Anthropological research showed that these patients had come from Egypt.[60] This is evidence of the development of a special order of pilgrimage which combined both religious and medicinal elements.[61] These reflected the successful integration of several conditions: the proximity to Jerusalem, the Biblical and Christian traditions related to the purification of people and curing of lepers in the waters of the Jordan[62] and the connection to the healing spas that dotted the entire Jordan Valley. By a carbon-14 dating conducted on the fragments of fabric found in the leper colony at the Monastery of John the Baptist, it appears that activity at the site should be dated to the ninth century.[63] Based on this, there is clear evidence of the continuity of the health services provided by the monks in the First Muslim Period following the Byzantine framework. This fact corresponds with information from the sixth-tenth centuries regarding the curing of lepers in the Dead Sea Basin. These sources refer explicitly to a cure marked by distinctly Christian elements which is attributed to the population

---

[55] On the Byzantine influence on the development of the Arab hospitals during the First Muslim Period, see: Hamarneh, p. 367.
[56] CCLS, p. 142; Wilkinson, p. 84.
[57] Wilkinson, pp. 137, 162.
[58] Zias, Garden, pp. 17-19.
[59] Theodosius, p. 36.
[60] Zias, Lepers, pp. 19-20; Zias, Disease, pp. 55-56.
[61] For more on this subject, see: Dvorjetski, Springs, p. 7-27.
[62] For example: the story of Na'aman in 2 Kings 5; John the Baptist, in John 26-28.
[63] Amar, Tradition, p. 28, note 21.

of greater Jerusalem and visitors to the area.[64] However, following the Arab conquest some of the monasteries were abandoned (some of the churches and monasteries had already been sacked during the Persian conquest in 614);[65] these were generally the monasteries situated in remote places. We have no evidence that these monasteries were abandoned due to a deliberate policy against religion enacted by the Muslims. Furthermore, there is evidence of the continued building of churches in the Jordan valley region from the beginning of the Muslim Period until the end of the Umayyad Period or until the beginning of the Abbasid Period.[66]

At any rate, the ramifications of the Arab conquest were indirect; and the abandonment of the monasteries, most of them small in size, may be explained by economic circumstances, a result of the absence of a policy of massive encouragement and support such as had been enjoyed previously under the Christian Byzantine government. On the other hand, one must note the continued existence of the large, major monasteries that were close to important border communities (Jerusalem, Bethlehem, and Jericho) where medical activity was concentrated. Among these monasteries are the Monastery of Theodosius, John the Baptist, Euthymius, Sabas, Gerasimus, and Haritun.[67] In other words, after the Arab conquest, one may speak of a certain decline in the volume of monastic activity which did however continue to function in the same patterns, adapting itself to the new political conditions that had been created. Furthermore, textual studies prove that in the period between the Muslim conquest and the Crusades, the monasteries of the Judean Desert continued to be centers vibrant with life and literary creativity[68], a factor that also greatly influenced medical science.

As we have seen, there is not much information available about the conventional medical tradition and methods in the Byzantine period as it was practiced in al-Sham and particularly in the Jerusalem region. Some of the information on physicians, methods of teaching medicine, and the medical curriculum may be learned from later sources. As to the status of the field of medicine, the First Muslim Period represents a direct continuation of the cultural and social reality of the Byzantine Period.

The First Muslim Period (640-1099)

New studies reveal that the land of Israel did not undergo a revolution in settlement and cultural patterns after the Muslim conquest in the seventh century. The Ummayad Period (660-750) is generally characterized by a uniformity and continuity of previous patterns of government. In the land of Israel during the First Muslim Period the solidly Byzantine Christian cultural foundations remained firmly in place, and are reflected in the material culture, as well as in the language, culture, and beliefs of the indigenous population.

[64] Amar. Tradition, pp. 27-28.
[65] See: Schick, Society, p. 83.
[66] Piccirillo, pp. 333-341; Schick, Christians, pp. 218-221; Schick, Society, pp. 207, 230.
[67] Hirschfeld, Monasteries, pp. 120-123.
[68] Griffith, pp. 57-78.

The studies show that in Greater Jerusalem, just prior to the Crusader conquest, there were still no clear-cut signs of Islamization, and the Christian influence remained powerfully predominant.[69]

Alongside the trend towards continuity of the spiritual and material culture that characterized the land of Israel in the period of transition between the Byzantine and Muslim periods, one must report on another process that applies to the Islamic world in its entirety. One of the most conspicuous changes that took place following the Islamic conquests is the cultural flowering in various fields of science in the Middle Ages. The Arabs, under whose control many cultures were unified, absorbed and adopted many branches of classical science and refined them. During the First Abbasid period (750-850 approx.) hundreds of medical manuscripts from different cultures, Greek-Roman and Syrian, were translated, documents that had been previously found in the pre-Islamic world. Especially noteworthy is the "Beit al-Hekama" translation project, founded in Baghdad by al-Maamun (813-833). The translation of classical sciences was carried out primarily by Christian translators who were a link between the two cultures. Original medical essays in Arabic also began to appear later. It seems that the convergence of all of these historical circumstances would readily explain the phenomenon of continuity of the local Byzantine medical tradition throughout the First Muslim Period.

Physicians, their status and medical training

We have no documentation on the physicians in Jerusalem and in the Land of Israel in general during the Ummayad Period (660-750). This may be related to the fact that the Muslim population was relatively small, and this did not require the planners of the Muslim regime to create a new system of public medicine. The lack of contact between the local physicians and the chroniclers of the period and their lack of contact and involvement with diplomatic and political process in the Islamic administration may have led to the lacuna in documentation on the subject. This is true also for the Abbasid Period which was centered in Baghdad; since that period the land of Israel became remote from the centers where Islamic policy was shaped.[70] Yet despite this, the influence of Arab centers of science slowly began to permeate the land of Israel as well.

Information about physicians in the Jerusalem region begin to appear in the tenth century. Medicine was still controlled by the Christians at that time as noted by the Jerusalem geographer al-Muqaddasi (985).[71] Sources on physicians in the Jerusalem region in this period are scant but even the little that is available confirms what al-Muqaddasi wrote. Two of the five physicians mentioned by name as being from Jerusalem are Christians who were considered worthy of being included in the essay on the history of medicine written by Ibn Abi Usaybia. The first was Yusef al-Nassrani, a prominent physician who was also familiar with other

[69] Amar, Islamization, pp. 249-252; Amar, Tradition, pp. 23-34; Klein-Franke, p. 105.
[70] Klein-Franke, pp. 111-112.
[71] Muqaddasi, p. 183.

sciences.[72] The second one was Zakariya Ibn Tuaba, a Jerusalem monk who also lived in the tenth century. Of the latter it has been said in general that he was very knowledgeable in the various sciences and in medicine. This physician was one of the teachers of the noted Muslim physician of Jerusalem, al-Tamimi.[73] From these sources it appears that medical learning in the land of Israel was still in the hands of the Christian monks, confined within the walls of the monasteries surrounding Jerusalem, and Muslims who wished to become proficient in the medical sciences were compelled to turn to them for knowledge. The monasteries in the land of Israel also contained valuable medical literature, some of which was written originally in Greek.[74] The chronicle of al-Tamimi's life also reveals that the study of medicine did not take place in an official academy but rather as study and apprenticeship under another qualified physician. We also know that his grandfather (but not his father) was a physician, so that it is possible that this was a profession taken up by certain families in the Jerusalem community.[75] This premise also suggests that the physicians enjoyed a high social standing and were connected to the ruling establishment. Yusef al-Nassrani was appointed by the Caliph Fatimid al-Áziz to be Patriarch of Jerusalem in 980 and al-Tamimi served initially in Ramla as personal physician to the governor Tkhshidi, al-Hassan ben Ábdallah ben Tghj. Later al-Tamimi moved to Egypt and was close to the vizier Ya'akub Ibn Killis (930-991), even writing a book for him.[76]

There were also Jewish physicians in Jerusalem. In the Geniza there is important information about a Jewish physician, a native of Jerusalem, who served as head of the Jewish community in the city.[77] In addition to this, physicians used to visit the city for short periods of time, among them one Gavriel ben Ábidalla ben Bakhtishua (d. 1007) who had the opportunity to visit Jerusalem for one day and then continued on to Damascus.[78]

The personality of al-Tamimi and his writings are a characteristic example of the portrayal of the unique local medical tradition that developed in our region over hundreds of years, on the one hand, and the development of an original Muslim medical tradition on the other. In his book, he cites information about materia medica, the way they were produced and used conventionally in the greater Jerusalem area. Especially interesting are the materia medica that originated in Jerusalem and environs. Al-Tamimi quotes in his essay many times from the Greek, Roman, and Byzantine medical authorities, such as: Aristotle, Dioscorides, Galenus and Paulus of Aegina (7th century). In addition he mentions the physicians from the "Period of the Translations" (ca. 750-850), such as Hunain b. Ishaq (809-877), and contemporary physicians

[72] Ibn Abi Usaybia, p. 545.
[73] Ibn Abi Usaybia, p. 546.
[74] Klein-Franke, pp. 112-113.
[75] On the biography of al-Tamimi, see: Ibn Abi Usaybia, pp. 546-548; Ibn al-Qifti, pp. 105-106; Amar, Tradition, pp. 23-25; Klein-Franke, pp. 115-117.
[76] Ibn Abi Usaybia, pp. 545-547.
[77] Goitein, Society, II, p. 257.
[78] Ibn Abi Usaybia, p. 213.

such as Ishaq al Israili (d, 953) and Ibn al-Jazar (920-1009).[79] It is clear that some of these essays were accepted and widespread as part of the medical studies in the Jerusalem region. At the same time, one must remember that some of his medical apprenticeship took place in Egypt and we have no way of knowing exactly which medical sources were available to him when he studied medicine in Jerusalem . In any case, it is clear that the source of the classical medical tradition that was practiced by the physicians in Jerusalem in the tenth century passed through two routes: through the Byzantine medical tradition, and beginning in the Abbasid Period was integrated and established in its Arab garb.

The production of theriac in Jerusalem and the trade in materia medica

Theriac is an anti-toxin serum produced from the venom of snakes, scorpions, and various components taken from the plant and mineral world. It appears that the technique of compounding theriac was a medical industry unique to the land of Israel in the Middle Ages and particularly during the First Muslim Period. Theriac is one of the most renowned medical preparations for which the land of Israel is celebrated as an export product. It is by deliberate choice that Rav Sa'adia Gaon (882-942) interpreted the "tzari" (Gen. 37:25, 43:11) which was sent "of the choice produce of the land" to Egypt as "theriac".[80]

This identification undoubtedly reflects the realia of his period. Many accounts, all of them from the tenth century, show that one of the most important centers for the production of theraic was Jerusalem.

At the end of the tenth century Rav Samuel ben Hofni Gaon wrote in his explication of the term "tzari" that "it referred to the Jerusalem theriac which was concocted of grasses in al-Sham and brought to different countries, and indeed it preserves the body from poisons".[81]

Al-Muqaddasi, a Jerusalem Moslem, also noted theriac among the products exported from Jerusalem.[82] In another place he notes that the city of Jericho was a source of snakes and scorpions (in another version "snakes and theriac"[83]) which were the major ingredients in preparing the theriac. [Fig. 8]

The literature refers to several well-known individuals who lived in Jerusalem in the tenth century and were engaged in the production of the theriac. Thus, for example, there is mention of a person whose very name is

[79] Amar, Tradition, pp. 23-34; all the descriptions of the land of Israel and an analysis of the sources of this author will be presented in a separate book currently being written by Z. Amar and Y. Seri.

[80] Kafik, on Gn. 37:25; Ibn Ezra on Gn. 37:25 added a paragraph in the name of Rav Saadiya Gaon that does not appear in his writings: "And the Gaon interpreted it as meaning that it was made up of 75 elements". On theraic, see fuller treatment in: Amar, Theraic.

[81] Greenbaum, on Gn. 43:11.

[82] Muqaddasi, p. 181.

[83] Muqaddasi, p. 173 as well as Mss. 14, c.

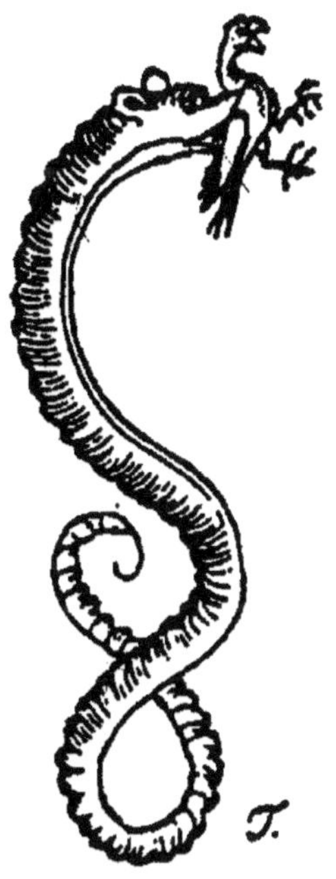

Figure 8: The 'Ter' snake from which the theriac was prepared in the Dead Sea region, as it is depicted in the work by Arnold von Harff, late fifteenth century.

testimony to his expertise: "Slama Ibn Nahatz al-Muqaddasi (of Jerusalem) al-Theriaqi.[84] However, more renowned for the production of theriac than any of these was the Jerusalem physician al-Tamimi. It is told of al-Tamimi that he had an extensive knowledge of medicine and was renowned for concocting salves and complex medicinal drugs. However, he achieved his greatest renown for his concoction of several varieties of theriac. We have information of at least four medical essays written by al-Tamimi on the subject of theriac: his large, intermediate, and small essay[85]. He also dedicated his letter (rassala) to his son Áli on the subject of "Theriac al-Faruq", which was held in great regard by the physicians of his day.

In addition to the fact that Jerusalem represented a concentration of experts possessing professional knowledge in combination with a center of production and export, the city also served as a source for supplying the individual ingredients used in making it. A considerable portion of the ingredients were made of plants, animals, and minerals from quarries which came from the Jerusalem region, and particularly from the Dead Sea basin which was connected administratively, economically, and culturally to the city of Jerusalem. Among the important ingredients in the compounding of theraic are asphalt and poisonous snakes which were hunted for this purpose in the Dead Sea region.[86]

The formulation of theriac from the venom of snakes in the region is explicitly mentioned in the essay of the pilgrim from Piacenza which was written circa 570.[87] In addition to that reference, we have an account of one of the monks of the Judean Desert who was bitten by a snake and taken by the residents of the village of Lazarion (al-Ázariya) close to Jerusalem to the hospital in the Holy City.[88] A physician and astrologist brought by the crusader king Amalric I (ruled 1162-1174) from Egypt to Jerusalem, used "Theriac al-Faruq" to treat King Amalric's son, Baldwin the Fourth, who was afflicted with leprosy.[89] Maimonides in his essay on theraic mentioned the herb "arqal-'haya" (identified as the Jerusalem fenugreek = Trigonella kotschyi) found in the Jerusalem region. "So did they give testimony that they saw him and his experience was

[84] Ibn al-Athir, al Lubab, p. 214.
[85] Ibn Abi Usaybia, pp. 546-548; Ibn al-Qifti, pp. 105-106.
[86] Amar, Theriac, pp. 22-24.
[87] CCLS, p. 136; Wilkinson, p. 82.
[88] Schwartz, p. 70.
[89] Ibn Abi Usaybia, p. 587-588, cf. : William of Tyre XXI, 1. During this period theraic was considered one of the most effective drugs against leprosy, see: Maimonides, Aphorisms, p. 147: "And eating the meat of a poisonous snake is a wonderful medication for those suffering from leprosy. And it should be eaten after its head and tail are cut off, its belly cleaned and washed out, and its skin removed. It should be cooked in much water and a little olive oil, dill, and leek, until soft.

verified… and in general a person would do well to have it prepared and to keep it by him at all times."[90] There is later testimony of the Jerusalem theriac from the eighteenth century, in a document itemizing the property of a Jew who had died.[91] Tobler reports in the middle of the nineteenth century that in the pharmacy belonging to Jews in Jerusalem one may find 'theriak'.[92] They tell that up until the present, there are descendants of the al-Theriaqi family in east Jerusalem who was engaged in collecting venom from snakes in the Jericho region.

As we have seen, theriac is one example of a drug containing many ingredients possessing healing properties which came from the area of Jerusalem and its environs. In addition to this, however, a wide variety of drugs was used in Jerusalem, which had been imported from great distances. Most of the information on this appears in letters from the eleventh century that were found in the Cairo Geniza and they attest to a lively trade in drugs originating in Egypt and North Africa.[93] Documents show that Jerusalem itself was an important way-station in the pharmaceutical trade, both domestic and foreign.[94] As part of the barter in various goods, perfumes and spices were also purchased that were in demand in Jerusalem.[95]

[90] Maimonides, Poisons, p. 107.
[91] Cohen, 18th Century, p. 482, note 65.
[92] Tobler, Medicine, p. 17.
[93] Gil, III, p. 165, no. 480; p. 173, no. 482.
[94] Gil, II, p. 421, no. 230.
[95] Gil, III, pp. 179-182, no. 485.

Chapter Four
The Crusader Period (until 1187)

The establishment of the Kingdom of Jerusalem (1099) began a new era in the history of the land of Israel. For some two hundred years (until 1291) the country was under Crusader rule, though the city of Jerusalem was governed without interruption by the Crusaders for only 88 years (until 1187). During this period, the religious significance of the Holy City increased in both the Christian and the Muslim world. The re-establishment of Jerusalem and its transfer to Christian rule with a western Christian orientation had vast implications for the city ideologically, economically, and socially. Extensive resources were directed towards the re-establishment of Jerusalem by Crusader policymakers. A tremendous human wave representing people from a different and unique stratum found its way to the city, among them: crusaders, merchants, soldiers, settlers, and clergy.[1]

An examination of the changes and influences on medicine in Jerusalem during the days of Crusader rule encounters many difficulties. Whereas there is abundant documentation during the Crusader period in comparison with the conspicuous dearth of material on the First Muslim Period, this documentation presents a narrow, single-faceted picture presented solely from the European point of view. This is provided by the Christian pilgrims or chroniclers who document the land of Israel from a religious world view which almost completely ignores the life and culture of the land of Israel. Thus there are still no clear-cut answers to many questions such as: What system of health services was available to the local population as a whole, and what happened to the hospitals which had been operated by the Eastern Christians? What kind of medicine in Jerusalem was practiced by the Franks? What was the source of inspiration for the hospital institution as established by the Hospitallers?

The status of medicine and sanitation in Jerusalem in the early Crusader Period

Before Jerusalem was captured by the Crusaders, a vast population had assembled between its walls, well beyond the city's capacity. Many refugees from the rural population, fearing the Crusader conquest, poured into the city. The chroniclers estimate that the city's population, which was twenty thousand people during peacetime, doubled and reached forty thousand, or according to one estimate, seventy thousand.[2] In addition, the Muslim general Iftikhar al-Daula had either stopped up the springs around Jerusalem or poisoned the waters, and this later caused a shortage of water for man and beast, both the besieged as well as the besiegers.[3] The hot climate inflicted many casualties upon the Crusaders who were unaccustomed to the regional conditions. Even before the conquest of Jerusalem, several of the Crusader leaders had contended

[1] Prawer, Jerusalem, pp. 29-32.
[2] William of Tyre VIII, 5: Ibn al-'Attir al-Kamil, X, p.283.
[3] Prawer, Kingdom, I, p. 136.

that due to the unbearable summer heat, the lack of water, shortage of horses, and the fatigue of the people as a result of famine, it would be sensible to postpone the campaign to capture Jerusalem until October when the weather was more suitable.[4] In the end, the campaign was conducted between June 7 and July 15 in 1099. During the siege many Crusader soldiers fell victim to heatstroke or died of thirst.[5] The crowded living conditions, lack of water and food, and faulty hygiene must have contributed to the outbreak and spread of disease among the Crusaders.[6] This problem was exacerbated by the Crusader conquest of Jerusalem. After five weeks of siege, the Crusaders conducted a massacre of the inhabitants of the city. Thousands of dead bodies piled up in the streets causing a terrible stench due to the summer heat. The Crusader leaders understood that the bodies could lead to the outbreak of epidemics and immediately set out on a campaign to cleanse the city of the corpses for fear of an outbreak of plague, as described by William of Tyre:

"The chiefs deemed it necessary, before all else, to cleanse the city, and especially the temple precincts, lest pestilence should arise from the air tainted by the stench from the corpses of the slain. This task was imposed upon those captured citizens who, though cast into prison, had by chance escaped death. But since their number was not sufficient to accomplish so great a work without aid, the poor of the army were offered a daily wage to give assistance in cleaning up the city without delay."[7]

The dead were buried at the foot of the eastern city wall. During the Crusader Period there were still several cemeteries located in various sites outside the walls of Jerusalem.[8] From the words of William of Tyre, it is not clear exactly who were those Crusader chiefs who were so mindful of the sanitation conditions of the city but it is known that as the kingdom became better established, there was a bourgeois court institution which took on the duty of policing the city and supervising the marketplaces and living arrangements in general. This institution possessed autonomous status and ultimate judicial authority. In this light, it is interesting to contemplate the story of the bourgeois citizens of Jerusalem who opposed and resisted the cleansing of the streets since one of the Crusader kings had ordered it done without them.[9]

Mortality from disease

There is scant information on the types of diseases and their mortality rates among the Crusaders,[10] while information about Jerusalem during the time of the first kingdom is even more scant. One may assume that even two generations after the Crusader conquest of Jerusalem there was still a prevalence of disease that claimed many casualties. According to the description of John of Würzburg (ca. 1165), some fifty out of two

---

[4] William of Tyre VII, 2.
[5] William of Tyre, VIII, 7.
[6] For a summary article on the diseases and sanitary conditions of the crusaders, see: Ficarra, pp. 135-155.
[7] William of Tyre, VIII, 24.
[8] Bahat, Topography, pp. 148-149.
[9] Prawer, Kingdom, I, p. 400, fn. 49.
[10] Ell, pp. 184-185; Ficarra, p. 140.

thousand people died every day in the hospitals established and operated by the Hospitallers, and their beds were immediately seized by new patients.[11] Even if one were to assume that this was an exaggerated estimate, it certainly contained a kernel of truth. It is not farfetched to assume that some of the patients who died succumbed to infectious diseases that spread within the hospital itself which supplied medical services to the hundreds of sick assembled there.

Most of the information that we have on the health conditions of the Crusaders in Jerusalem refers to a description of the diseases suffered by the Crusader chiefs, and this may shed light to some extent on the nature of the diseases that were common at that time. From the examples brought here we may see that the life expectancy of the Crusader kings was generally short. Godfrey of Bouillon (1099-1100) was afflicted with a severe disease which became more serious from day to day; efforts to find an effective cure were futile, and he died.[12] His brother Baldwin I (1100-1118), the first to be crowned "King of Jerusalem", was wounded by a spear near Tyre. Thanks to treatment by his physicians, he recovered, yet periodically suffered pain from the wound which had never totally healed. His sickness overcame him and he eventually succumbed to it near El-'Arish (Sabhat Bardawil). [13] Baldwin II (1118-1131) was overcome by a severe illness while in Jerusalem[14], and his grandson Baldwin III (1143-1162) was 33 when he died of sickness.[15] He recalls that he had apparently been poisoned by his physician in Antioch when he took a physic before the approach of winter. The mother of Baldwin III, Queen Melisenda (1131-1152) fell ill of an incurable disease which affected her memory and weakened her body. She lay in this helpless situation for a long time before dying in 1161.[16] King Amalric I (1162-1174) was afflicted with dysentery and fever and died, apparently of cholera.[17] Amalric's son, Baldwin IV (1174-1185) was afflicted with leprosy and died while still a young man.[18] King Baldwin V died in 1186 at the age of eight. [Fig. 9]

These are just several examples of famous personages from the Crusader world who were active in Jerusalem, and most of them met their death there. A comparison of the life expectancy for the Crusader aristocracy in general shows a similarly short life expectancy.[19] The explanation for this is related to the faulty sanitation and the prevalence of infectious diseases. It is possible that in some cases, these were diseases that the Crusaders brought with them from Europe[20] that were not common or familiar in the east, so that local medicine was unable to provide the proper medical solution.

---

[11] PPTS V, p. 44.
[12] William of Tyre, IX, 23.
[13] William of Tyre, X, 26; X, 31.
[14] William of Tyre, XIII, 28.
[15] William of Tyre, XVIII, 34.
[16] William of Tyre, XVIII, 27.
[17] William of Tyre, XX, 31. According to Tobler, Medicine, p. 45, he died of dysentery.
[18] William of Tyre, XXI, 1; XXII, 9; XXII, 25.
[19] Prawer, History, p. 256.
[20] Ficarra, p. 142.

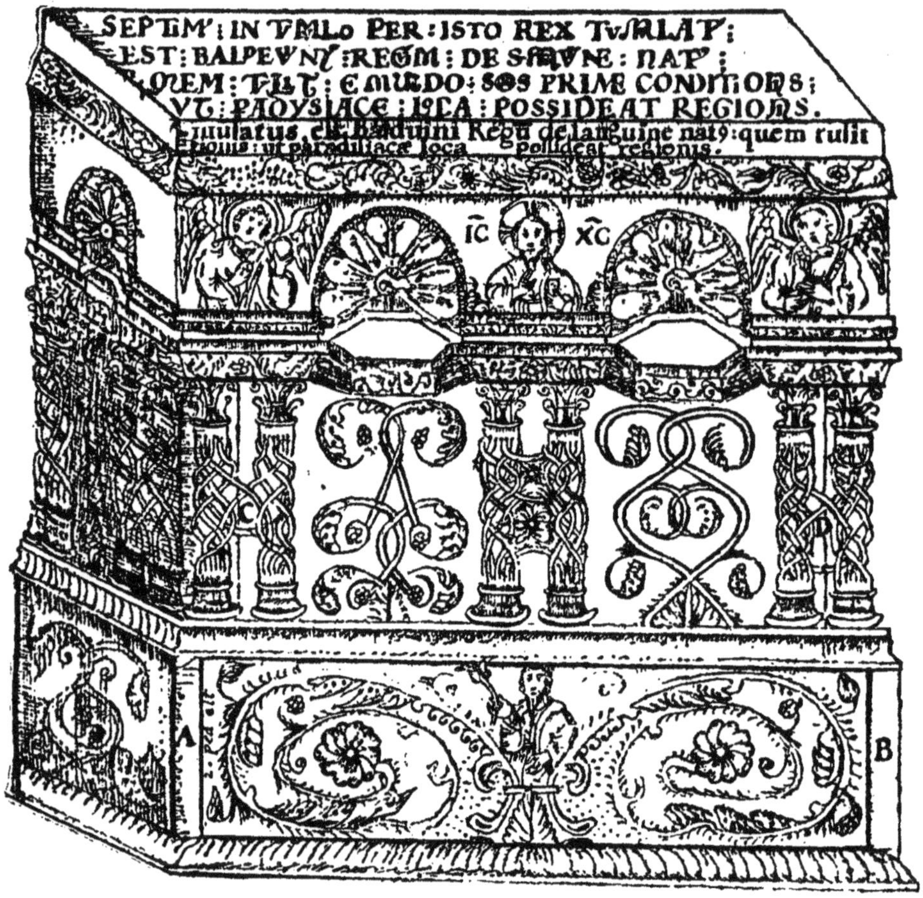

Figure 9: Gravestone of Baldwin V, who died in 1186 at the age of eight.

It is worth noting that all of the examples cited here are provided by William of Tyre, the chronicler of the Crusader Period. He was born in the Crusader Kingdom of Jerusalem in 1127, apparently in Jerusalem proper, to parents of European birth, and he died ca. 1185. He was close to the royal court and served as tutor to Baldwin IV. William of Tyre had enjoyed a liberal education and apparently was not a stranger to medical literature. In his writing, one may find vast medical information meticulously described, and in the case of the leprosy of Baldwin IV, he even quotes the precise description of the disease according to Hippocrates.[21] In William of Tyre's essay one may also find something else symbolic, that is worth quoting in the context of mortality from disease. As opposed to the Frankish rulers, the Muslim ruler Nur al-Din appears as the only sick person who recovered from what was described as an incurable disease, but his recovery took place thanks to the devoted treatment of the physicians of the Orient.[22] Does this suggest the superiority of local medicine over Frankish medicine?

[21] William of Tyre, XXI, 1.

[22] William of Tyre, XVII, 17-21. Incidentally, Nur al-Din (1118-1174) was fifty six years old when he died of a disease of the throat (tonsilitis or diphtheria), see: Ibn al-'Attir, al-Kamil, XI, p. 402; El s.v. Nur al-Din.

The Medical Services of the Eastern Christians

After the Crusader conquest, there were scarcely any Jews or Muslims left in Jerusalem. Most had been massacred, some had been taken captive, and the rest fled.[23] The local Christian population who had been expelled from Jerusalem by the Muslims before the start of the Crusaders' siege returned to the city after it was captured by the Crusaders.

The Eastern Christian population in its various divisions was accorded neither sympathetic nor equal treatment by the Crusaders. This was the result of religious and cultural differences. Religiously, the Crusaders were closely attached to the center of Roman-Catholicism in Rome rather than to Eastern Orthodoxy. The Eastern Orthodox population which had undergone a process of intermingling during the years of Muslim rule was in effect part of the Eastern culture. The local Christians adopted the material and spiritual life-style of the Arabs: the Arabic language, foods, garb, etc. In that respect they were very different from the western Franks in their customs and culture and more like the Muslims. Thus the Crusaders treated them with suspicion, openly displaying their contempt. The status of the Eastern Christians was inferior and there is actually no evidence of the Franks showing a preferential attitude toward the Christians over the non-Christians. Furthermore, some of the assets of the Eastern Greek church were confiscated and transferred to representatives of the Latin clergy or the aristocratic laity who treated the Christians as an occupied population. What emerges then is that the Crusaders followed a policy of discrimination of the Eastern Christians who were denied positions in state and government and even in the Church.[24]

We have scarcely any information about the medical services available to the local Christian population of Jerusalem and the environs in the Crusader period. However, the attitude of the Franks to the Eastern Christians can lead us to surmise that there was a separation between Frankish medical services and those of the local population. A second assumption is that the healing institutions of the local population were largely based on the infrastructure that had survived from the Byzantine and First Muslim periods.

During the Crusader Period, the Eastern Church preserved its monastic character, both in its social structure and in its worldview.[25] It also succeeded in preserving part of its institutions and properties in the villages and monasteries outside of Jerusalem. Around Jerusalem most of the Judean Desert monasteries continued to exist as they had during Muslim rule, for instance, the Mar Elias, Theodosios, and Mar Saba monasteries, and they continued the practices of the ancient charter outlined by Basil.[26] For lack of alternate medical institutions, the Eastern Christian church continued to provide medical services to the local population,

[23] Prawer, Kingdom, I, pp. 141-142; Prawer, Jerusalem, pp. 22-24.
[24] Prawer, Colonial, pp. 232-234, 578-579; Rose, pp. 176-181.
[25] Rose, p. 177.
[26] Prawer, Colonial, pp. 239-242.

Christian and Muslim alike. This assertion is reinforced by information about the functioning of these institutions during the Ayyubid Period, as will be seen in following. One example of this is the hospital that had been at the Mar Saba monastery, even though it is possible that during this time it was controlled by the Latin Church in Jerusalem.[27]

Medical services of the Frankish Christians

In contrast to the paucity of information on medicine among the local population, there is much documentation on the Crusader medical institutions in Jerusalem and how they operated. However, the information almost entirely describes the medical services provided by the military orders who offered this service, primarily to the Crusaders.

From the beginning of the thirteenth century we find suggestions that the Order of Hospitallers was also giving medical service to members of the upper class, among them the nobility and churchmen. From this, Nilsson & Sunzel seek to deduce that all strata of the population of all social classes and nationalities were dependent on the hospital services provided by the Hospitallers, rather than on private medicine.[28] However we have no evidence from the numerous sources which describe the hospital in Jerusalem (until it was conquered by Saladin in 1187), that it did indeed treat the sick who were neither Crusaders, the indigent, nor members of the order. On the contrary, what these sources show is that the Hospitallers made it their declared objective to treat the Crusaders and the indigent, and not to provide a solution for public medicine.[29] Only in one document (from before 1187) is there any mention of the term "the sick" in a general way, without singling out the Crusaders and the indigent. However, this document refers to the hospital in Acre, not Jerusalem.[30] In other words, it is hard to infer the later reality that evolved in the Kingdom of Jerusalem after the Battle of the Horns of Hattin (1187) where subsequently the institution of medicine in Jerusalem had to undergo modifications in functioning, from the golden age of the institution on the eve of the Muslim conquest.[31]

[27] Richard, p. 91. fn.8.

[28] Nilsson & Sunzel, p. 15.

[29] Kedar,(Hospital, p. 7) cites an anonymous source which notes that the hospital served the entire population, with no distinction of gender or race, including Jews and Muslims. However, it seems that this was a theoretical declaration taken from the medical statutes, such as those of Salerno (see: **Sterns**) and that it was not actually practiced at the St. John's Hospital in Jerusalem. In practice, even if Jews also had been allowed to receive medical treatment at the hospital , it is doubtful that they would have availed themselves of this, for beginning with the admittance procedure, the hospital stay included unmistakably Christian religious symbols which, Jews loyal to their faith, were unable to accept in any form. The statement that appears in the Statutes of the Order of 1182 according to which patients who are unable to eat pork would receive chicken (Hospitaller documents no. 627, p. 428), in my opinion, was not directed at the Jewish or Muslim patients bur rather a statute that relates to the personal preferences or physical requirements (e.g. digestive status) of each patient.

[30] For example, in all of the statutes and grants, the hospital was designated to serve the pilgrims and the poor, see i.e.: Hospitaller documents, no. 30, pp. 29-30; no. 47, pp. 39-40; no. 130, p. 107; no. 246, pp. 185-186; nos. 203-204, p. 270.

[31] Hospitaller documents, no. 471, pp. 323-324, from 1175 CE.

We are also lacking information about the hostel services which included medical treatment under the auspices of the institutions of the Latin Church in Jerusalem. In contrast, there is evidence of treatment for the sick pilgrims who visited the Church of the Nativity in Bethlehem, near Jerusalem. While this information refers to a later period, namely the middle of the thirteenth century, it would still appear that the organization of the hospital institution which was subject to the Patriarch of Jerusalem actually was earlier.[32] But there, too, the target audience was limited to pilgrims and the indigent. The foregone conclusion is that there were additional medical institutions that gave service to the large Frankish community in Jerusalem, which included settlers, merchants, and nobility. We have no information about the establishment of a government-sponsored hospital, and it would seem that most medical therapy was carried out in the private sector, by Frankish or eastern Christian physicians who practiced in their homes. Examples of Frankish physicians who lived in Jerusalem and even acquired property there are: Roberto the physician and William the physician.[33] It is hard to estimate the dimensions of this phenomenon but it must have been prevalent among the wealthy.

Members of the aristocracy and the royal family employed the services of private physicians of great repute. Physicians were summoned periodically to treat these people, but there were those who had personal physicians who received a regular salary for their work. In this sense, the Frankish rulers adopted the practice of "the court physicians" which had been widely accepted among the Muslims in their day. An interesting example of this is the Egyptian physician, Abu Suliman Daud b. Abi al-Mana b. Abi Fana who was brought by the Crusader king Amalric (ruled 1162-1174) to Jerusalem with his five children. One of Abu Suliman's sons grew up and was educated in Jerusalem together with Baldwin IV and became a Crusader knight, while his four other sons practiced medicine in the service of various Ayyubid rulers. Abu Suliman treated Baldwin IV, the son of Amalric, who was afflicted with leprosy.[34] It is quite clear that Amalric, like the kings, used the services of other physicians. William of Tyre recounts, apropos the treatment of Baldwin IV: "The lad's father was informed of his condition, and physicians were consulted. Repeated fomentations, oil rubs, and even poisonous remedies were employed without result in the attempt to help him."[35]

In Jerusalem one could find physicians from the East as well as Frankish physicians. When King Amalric fell ill and began to suffer from dysentery as he approached Tiberias, he feared that the disease would overwhelm him and he continued on through Nazareth and Nablus to Jerusalem. There he summoned Greek and Syrian physicians, as well as medical practitioners of other nationalities. When, for professional reasons, they refused to give him the drugs that he demanded, he called in Frankish physicians.[36] Expert physicians

---

[32] Richard, p. 95.
[33] Röhricht, Regesta, document. no. 170, p. 42 (from 1137 CE); nos.430-431, p. 112 (from 1167); no. 182, p. 45 (from 1138).
[34] Ibn abi Usaybi'a, pp. 587-589.
[35] William of Tyre, XXI, 1.
[36] William of Tyre, XX, 31.

were also called in to treat Queen Melisenda who fell ill of an incurable disease, and they assiduously applied such remedies as were judged most effective.[37]

Another example of the fact that one could find excellent medical services in Jerusalem was the following event: When Baldwin I was wounded in an incident with pirates in Tyre in 1103, he returned to Jerusalem knowing that there he would find skillful physicians who could treat him. William of Tyre notes that "the care of the physicians, however, with their use of incisions and cautery at length restored Baldwin to some degree of health…".[38]

The medical services of the military orders

The military orders are an original creation of the Crusader Kingdom. These orders were guided by an ideology that fused knightly warrior strength with the monastic ideals as forged by the Templars. The major purpose for which the orders were originally established was to care for the pilgrims and to protect the roads leading to the holy sites. Later, the orders undertook clearly military functions which were an important and significant component in defending the Crusader kingdom.[39] We will not deal with this aspect at present. The double task undertaken by the knights is described by Rabbi Benjamin of Tudela who visited Jerusalem ca. 1170: "The city also contains two buildings, from one of which – the hospital – there issue forth four hundred knights; and therein all the sick who come thither are lodged and cared for in life and in death".[40]

The most important military orders which were involved in providing medical service in Jerusalem were the Hospitallers, its German branch (later known as the Teutonic Knights), and the Knights of St. Lazarus. The Templar order was of a more pronouncedly military character and its charter contains much information which largely relates to the care of sick knights.[41] The Hospitallers may serve as a prototype of the activity of the orders which developed the practice of medicine in Jerusalem, whose declared purpose was to care for the indigent and sick and about which there is relatively scant available information.

The Order of Hospitallers

The beginning of the Order of Hospitallers may be seen as a philanthropic institution founded in Jerusalem at the incentive of Italian merchants from Amalfi in the middle of the eleventh century. The Amalfitans established an inn and hospital (Hospitum) for pilgrims from Europe in the area of the Muristan in the

---

[37] William of Tyre, XVIII, 27.
[38] William of Tyre, X, 26.
[39] Prawer, Kingdom, I, pp. 388-398; Prawer, Colonial, pp. 330-357.
[40] Adler, pp. 22.
[41] See e.g. : The Templars Rule, nos. 190-197, pp. 65-66. For the medical treatment of knights, see: Sterns, pp. 43-69.

Christian Quarter.[42] Some scholars date this to an earlier time and believe that they actually rehabilitated the building and philanthropic projects of Charlemagne (ca. 800) which had been destroyed during the time of the caliph, al-Hakim (1009). The attempt to identify these buildings is problematic and controversial.[43] The hospital which belonged to the Hospitallers is thus the continuation of the Amalfitans' hospital, and is referred to in the beginning of the Crusader period. The first account is the reference by Saewulf who visited Jerusalem in 1102[44], even before the Crusaders had managed to leave their imprint on the city. Gerard, a knight from the south of France, served as administrator of the hospital until 1120. With the Crusader conquests of Jerusalem, the institution flourished and became one of the city's central public institutions. In 1113 the Order and the Jerusalem hospital were accorded recognition by Pope Paschal II. The Order enjoyed many privileges, among them exemption from paying the church tithe, and this gave the Order an independent status and released it from the discipline of the local church hierarchy.[45]

The knights of the Order were first named for John the Almoner, the patriarch of Alexandria in the seventh century. As the institution developed and brought with it a change in the character of the Order, its patron was also replaced and it was dedicated to Saint John the Baptist. In approximately 1130 Fetellus makes note of the inn and the hospital (infirmorum) at the St. John the Baptist Church complex.[46] William of Tyre also mentions the Hospitallers' medical establishment which provided for the pilgrims, where the sick were accommodated and the indigent and homeless were given food and shelter.[47]

The St. John's Hospital and the adjacent church were located in the Patriarch's quarter known until today as Muristan. This is a distortion of the Persian term 'bimaristan' meaning 'hospital' which made its way into the Arabic name. The contemporary sources mention the building and its location, but the descriptions are not uniform, and in modern research, there is no agreement over the precise location of the building. Remnants of the building are generally considered to be located in the assembly room of the Omarya Mosque.[48] Descriptions of pilgrims who visited the site at a later period speak of a vast, domed building which contained many rooms. [49] The St. John's Hospital of the Hospitallers appears in medieval maps of Jerusalem, [Fig. 10] and of particular interest, in the Codex Harleian which calls it "the pilgrims' hospital".[50]

The hospital institution received a significant impetus to its development under the leadership of Raymond du Puy, the second Master of the Order (1120-1160) who in his day transformed the order into a

[42] King, pp. 11-12; Miller, Birth, p. 728; Richard, pp. 89-90.

[43] See Prawer, Kingdom, pp. 389-390; Bahat, Layout, p. 48-52, 77, fn. 356.

[44] In: PPTS IV, p. 14.

[45] Hospitaller documents, I, no. 30, p. 29; for more about the other privileges and grants accorded the Hospitallers, see: Nilsson & Sunzel, p. 12.

[46] Fetellus, PPTS, V, p. 2.

[47] William of Tyre, XVIII, 5.

[48] For a discussion of the location of the hospital complex, see: Delaville, pp. 28-29; Bahat, Topography, pp. 86-91; Patrich, Structure, pp. 3-16; Schein, pp. 148-150; Burgoyne, p. 568.

[49] Schein, pp. 147-148.

[50] Levy, Maps, pp. 427, 475.

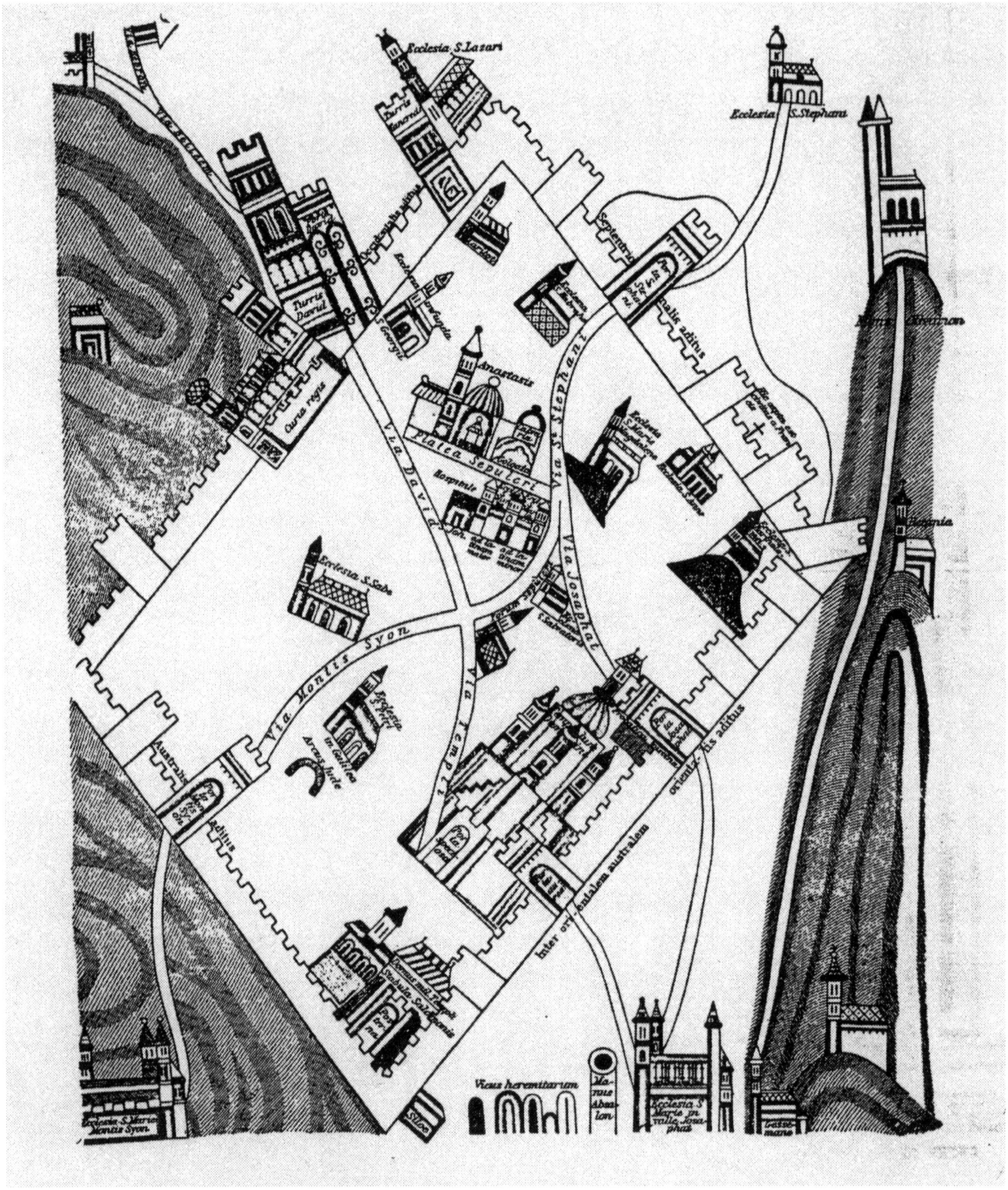

Figure 10: Map of Crusader-controlled Jerusalem in the 12th century (Cambrai Map): north of the city (outside the walls) one can discern the Church of Lazarus and nearby the leprosarium. Within the walls, beyond the Plaza of the Holy Sepulcher (Platea Sepulcri) is the St. John's Hospital (S. Johannis Hospitale).

major political and military factor.[51] During his time, apparently between 1130-1140, the hospital was rebuilt and expanded.[52] It reached its peak of development and organization under the appointment of Roger des Moulins, Master of the Order of Hospitallers (1177-1187).[53] The institution provided service to the thousands of pilgrims who visited Jerusalem, especially the indigent and sick who could not afford the private medical services which were for hire. The hospital was described with much wonder by the many pilgrims who came to the city. Rabbi Benjamin of Tudela states thus: "And therein all the sick who come thither are lodged and cared for in life and in death."[54] There are two more important descriptions from the seventh decade of the twelfth century relating to the location and function of the building. John of Würzberg writes in his essay of ca. 1165 as follows:

> "Over against the Church of the Holy Sepulchre, which we have described above, on the opposite side (of the way), towards the south, is a beautiful church built in honour of John the Baptist, annexed to which is a hospital, wherein in various rooms is collected together an enormous multitude of sick people, both men and women, who are tended and restored to health daily at a very great expense. When I was there I learned that the whole number of these sick people amounted to two thousand, of whom sometimes in the course of one day and night more than fifty are carried out dead, while many other fresh ones keep continually arriving. What more can I say? This same house supplies as many outside with victuals as it does those inside, in addition to the boundless charity which is daily bestowed upon poor people who beg their bread from door to door and do not lodge in the house, so that the whole sum total of its expenses can surely never be calculated even by the managers and stewards thereof."[55]

From this description one can see that this was a building with a large capacity to accommodate the massive number of pilgrims who required its services. According to John of Würzburg, the house had a high mortality rate and this is evidence of the poor state of health and the faulty hygiene that prevailed in Jerusalem, and it appears that even this hospital was unable to meet all of the medical needs that arose. The hospital institution handled not only the sick but also served as a soup kitchen for the needy. More complete information about the structure of the hospital and the source of the considerable funding required to keep it operating may be found in the description given by Theodorich from ca. 1172:

> "...and here, on the south side of the church, stands the Church and Hospital of Saint John the Baptist. As for this, no one can credibly tell another how beautiful its buildings are, how abundantly it is supplied with rooms and beds, and other material for the use of the poor and sick, ... Indeed, we

[51] Miller, Knights, p. 718.
[52] King, p. 12.
[53] Nilsson & Sunzel, pp. 14-15.
[54] Adler, p. 22.
[55] PPTS, V, p. 44.

> passed through this palace, and were unable by any means to discover the number of sick people lying there; but we saw that the beds numbered more than one thousand. It is not everyone even of the most powerful kings and despots who could maintain as many people as that house does every day; and no wonder, for, in addition to its possessions in other countries (whose sum total is not easily to be arrived at), the Hospitallers and the Templars have conquered almost all the cities and villages which once belonged to Judaea…"[56]

Both descriptions note the large number of sick people; one mentions two thousand patients while the second notes over a thousand beds. Some scholars resolve the discrepancy between the two estimates by the fact that in the House of the Sick run by the Hospitallers, two patients shared one bed, apparently the standard practice in Europe.[57] [Fig. 11] Possible support for this explanation may be seen in the seal of the Templar order which shows two knights riding on the same horse, and this is explained as a symbol of the poverty associated with the Order. [Fig. 12][58] It seems that the hospital was planned to accommodate approximately one thousand people in times of calm. This number is also cited by the pilgrims visiting the site during the Mamluk period, when it was used only as an inn.[59] However, during emergencies, for example during an outbreak of epidemic, the hospital was forced to accommodate a larger number. When the hospital reached capacity, the knights of the order had to give up their beds on behalf of the sick.[60] Moreover, the hospital did not limit its care to the pilgrims and the indigent but also supplied medical care to the wounded who were sent there from the battles between the Muslims and the Crusaders. Jerusalem and the areas that controlled the roads leading to it became a battlefield and a constant target of attack. The hospital's ability to admit hundreds of the wounded is attested to by the Battle of Tel Djezer (Montgisart) in November of 1177. At that time, Jerusalem stood in real danger of conquest by the Muslims. It is told that in the hospital run by the Hospitallers, the sick were even taken out of their beds, in order to kneel together with the knights of the Order and to hold prayers for the salvation of the city.[61] The pressure of contemplating future events must have caused the hospital officials to make the necessary preparations. Eventually the Muslim army suffered a painful defeat which also exacted a heavy price among the Crusaders. It is recorded that seven hundred and fifty casualties were sent for treatment at the hospital, in addition to the nine hundred who were already being cared for there.[62] In an event of that kind, the surgeons who were part of the medical staff of the hospital came into play, and their assignment was to treat the casualties of battle.[63] The surgeons were positioned close to the battlefield and offered help to the wounded. Those who required additional treatment were sent to Jerusalem on camels, horses, mules, and donkeys that belonged to the Order. If there was a lack

[56] PPTS, V, p. 22.
[57] Bahat, Topography, p. 91, fn. 152.
[58] Prawer, Epigraphy, p. 387.
[59] See: Ludolph Von Suchem (1341), in: PPTS, XII, pp. 106-107; Felix Fabri (1483), in: PPTS VII-VIII, p. 395.
[60] Adington, Hospital, p. XIII.
[61] Prawer, Kingdom, I, p. 445.
[62] Röhricht, Articles, II, pp. 127-128.
[63] Adington, Hospital, p. XIV.

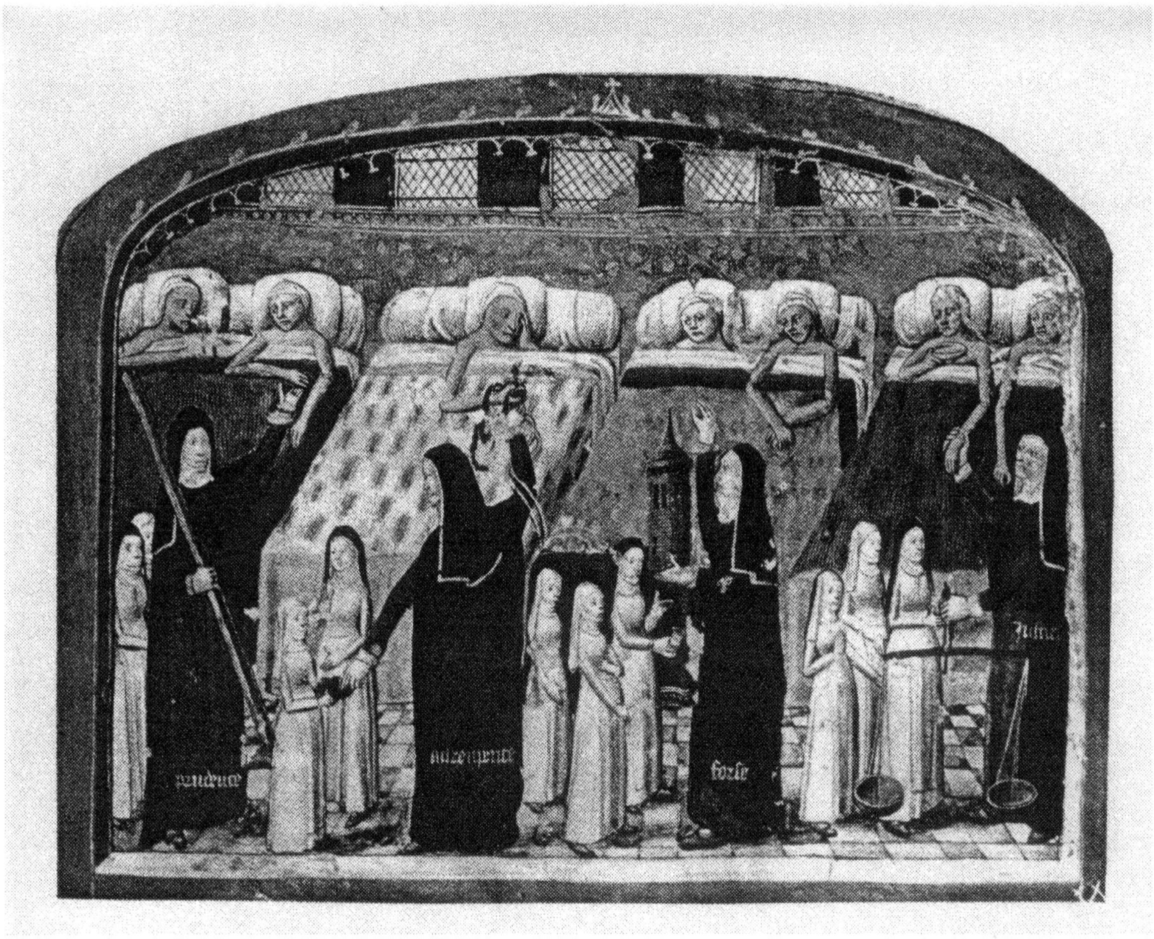

Figure 11: Medieval women's hospital, where two patients shared one bed. Standing in front of the beds are the staff of nursing brothers and sisters. (Morris, p. 178)

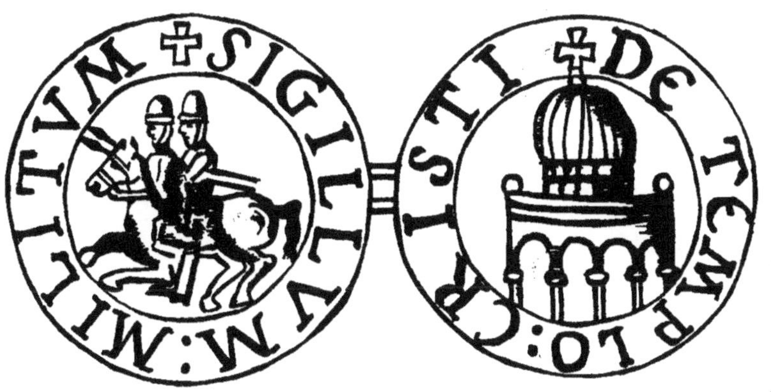

Figure 12: Seal of the Order of Templars.

of beasts of burden, the knights of the order hired additional animals or dismounted their own horses and placed the wounded on their backs. This was an example of the well-developed system for evacuating the wounded that characterizes military medicine. Kedar notes that this was a system unparalleled in Catholic Europe of that time whence the Hospitallers had come. In contrast, a similar system did exist in the Islamic world.[64]

Care of the sick

Most of the information on treatment of the sick and the organization of the hospital comes to us from two types of sources, from the seventh and eighth decade of the twelfth century. The first type is the literature written by the pilgrims, and of particular note, the anonymous pilgrim who received treatment at the hospital and incidentally recorded his impressions.[65] The second type is the Statutes of the Order in Jerusalem, particularly in the days of Roger des Moulin, Master of the Order of Hospitallers (1177-1187), which represents a new era in the life of the Order. There are two versions of the statutes which supplement each other and also shed light on the other sources.[66] It should be noted that in these statutes there is no mention of any military type of activity, which implies that the inspiration for writing them was not original, but rather had been copied from a different, clearly medical charter. According to Sterns, they show a strong influence of the Salerno Medical School.[67]

We learn of the patient admittance process in one of the statutes of Raymond du Puy, the second Master of the Order from the mid-twelfth century, who discusses the procedure: "How should our lords – the patients - be accepted and be served?". After the patient received permission from one of the heads of the Order to make use of the hospital's services, he would take part in the prayer service and undergo confession with the priest. Then he would be carried to his bed and be given food, depending on the supply available at the time.[68] The patient admittance process also included a meticulous registering and safekeeping of his personal effects. His personal possessions and arms were stored in a warehouse (karavane); his clothes were placed in a sack and his money was put into safekeeping. The warehouse would be opened twice a year or more, and the patients were called upon to identify their possessions. There were clear orders regarding a situation where the sack of clothes was lost, as well as instructions for transferring possessions as a religious trust to the Order, in the event that the patient died without any heirs.[69] This procedure was undoubtedly influenced by the military nature of the Order and was designed to guarantee the existence of a standardized public system and to prevent exploitation and injury to the helpless sick.

---

[64] Kedar, Hospital, p. 7.
[65] Adington, Hospital; Kedar, Hospital.
[66] Nilsson & Sunzel, pp. 14-15; Adington, Hospital, p. X.
[67] Sterns, pp. 45, 54-55.
[68] Hospitaller documents, no. 70, p. 67, dated between 1125 and 1153, chap. 16; see also: Nilsson & Sunzel, pp. 12-13; Miller, Knights, p. 718; Hume, p. 28.
[69] Adington, Hospital, p. XII.

The Rule of the Order also details the personal equipment issued to each patient, which includes a bed, bedsheets, and clothing. Thus, for example, it was determined in the directions of the order that the patients' beds must be long and wide enough so that they are suitable for comfortable reclining, and that every bed must be covered with its own coverlet and equipped with its own set of sheets. Likewise, it was decreed that little cradles should be made for the babies of women pilgrims who are born in the hospital, so that they might lie separate. Every patient was to be given the following items of clothing: a cloak of sheepskin, boots for walking to the latrines, and a woolen cap.[70]

One can learn how the hospitals operated from the following excerpt:

> "The Holy House of the Hospital is accustomed to receive sick men and women and is accustomed to keep doctors who have care of the sick and who make syrups for the sick, and who provide the things that are necessary for the sick. For three days in the week, the sick are accustomed to have fresh meat, either pork or mutton, and those who are unable to eat it have chicken.
> And two sick persons are accustomed to have one cloak of sheep-skin (*pelice de brebis*) which they use when going to the latrines (*chambres)* and between two sick persons, one pair of boots. Every year the House of the Hospital is accustomed to give to the poor one thousand cloaks of thick lamb skins.
> And all the children abandoned by their fathers and mothers, the House of the Hospital is accustomed to receive and to nourish. To a man and woman who desire to enter into matrimony, and who possess nothing with which to celebrate the marriage, the House of the Hospital is accustomed to give two bowls (*escueles*) or the rations of two brethren..."[71]

As to the subject of abandoned children, it emerges from the tale of an anonymous writer that this was a common phenomenon; poor women would leave their infants at the Hospital door. There were also women who gave birth to twins and would leave one of the newborns at the hospital. The foundlings were entrusted to nurses who were hired by the hospital at the rate of 12 gold coins per year. These foundlings were known all over the Frankish Orient as "the children of John the Baptist" and when they reached puberty, they could decide whether to join the Order or to lead regular secular lives.[72]

These sources show that the hospital did not just treat the sick but also served as a philanthropic institution supplying all of the needs of the poor and needy, as was accepted practice in Europe until the sixteenth century.[73] The text depicts a portrait of severe human misery which even this institution could scarcely relieve, to the extent where every two patients had to share the most basic items that had been given. Another

---

[70] Hospitaller documents, no. 627, p. 426.
[71] Hospitaller documents, no. 627, pp. 426-428.
[72] Kedar, Hospital, p. 7.
[73] Seidler, pp. 2-22.

example of this may be seen in a document from 1176 which quotes the decision of the head of the Order of Hospitallers, that white bread (*pain blanc)* is one of the privileges granted the sick in the hospital in Jerusalem. This bread had to be of a certain weight and was divided between two people. Buying bread for the sick was financed by income from the villages of 'Abud (S.Marie) and Caphaer in the southern hills of Samaria.[74]

Patients were also served twice a day, morning and evening, wine or a sweetened beverage (depending on the patient's preference).[75] It is noteworthy that the white bread and wine were considered food possessing great medicinal properties at that time in Arab medicine in the east.[76] Of special note is the use of sugar as a sweetener in the medicinal compounds concocted in the hospital. In the Rule of the Order, it is mentioned in connection with "syrop"[77], a term that the Franks borrowed from the word "rubb" in Arabic. A similar term 'sharab' means 'drink', and in medical terminology, refers to a medicinal beverage generally made of fruit juice, cooked and sweetened with sugar. The Crusaders must have learned the medicinal use of sugar only in the land of Israel for it had yet to be used in Western Europe.[78] Sugar, then, is an example par excellence of the Crusaders' adopting some of the local medical substances in the land of Israel, and from there, transferring it to Europe. This was possible because some of the physicians at the hospitals operated by the Hospitallers were easterners and also because of the more readily availability of these materia medica. Another basic medicinal foodstuff in use at the hospital was almonds, used to prepare almond milk, which was served regularly as part of the weekly diet.[79] Using almonds and sugar as medicinal products is also mentioned in Jerusalem during the Ayyubid Period.[80]

In another version of the Rule of the Order, there is an itemization of the kinds of meat that were supplied at the hospital, depending on the season of year: chicken, goats, lambs, and pork if the physicians so instructed. During the fast of Lent, fish was given three times a week, as well as cooked vegetables and vegetable soup. Beyond the fixed menu, other foods were occasionally given: eels, cheese, lentils, beans, and cabbage. The sick also received three fruits such as: pomegranates, apples, pears, plums, figs, and grapes.[81]

In short the menu was devised so as to raise the patients' intake of calories and vitamins and to strengthen them. Beyond the basic foodstuffs and medicines, such as bread, wine, sugar, and meat, there is almost no listing of any other medicinal substances or prescriptions, apparently because a wide range of medicines was given, based on the medical methods and training and professional literature, which may have varied from

---

[74] Hospitaller documents, no. 494, pp. 339-340.
[75] Adington, Hospital, p. XI. Spiced wine is an important ingredient in the medical statutes of Salerno, see; Sterns, p. 59.
[76] White bread and wine are mentioned in the medical guide written by Maimonides for al-Iafdal, the son of Saladin, see: Maimonides, Regimen, p. 35, fns. 38, 87.
[77] Hospitaller documents, no. 627, pp. 426-427.
[78] See: Amar, Innovations, pp. 89-91.
[79] Adington, Hospital, p. XI.
[80] Goitein, Jewry, p. 324.
[81] Adington, Hospital, p. X; a similar diet is mentioned in the Salerno charter, see: Sterns, p. 54.

one physician to the next.[82] However, we are also lacking information about the methods used to diagnose the various diseases and the nature of treatment given. The only specific mention of medical treatment appears in the context of those wounded in battle, where general reference is made to the use of plants and minerals. Use of these materials was accepted practice throughout the medical world in the Middle Ages, part of the tradition of Dioscordes (first century).[83]

Separate treatment for men and women

In a document cited previously, it is explicitly mentioned that " the House of the Hospital was accustomed to receive sick men and women". It is patently clear that there was a total separation between men and women. Moreover, women whose husbands were hospitalized were not permitted to stay with their husbands and they were lodged separately in a hall adjacent to the hospital.[84]

Parallel to the Hospitaller's activity in the hospital, there is mention of another hospital in Jerusalem for women, that was named for Saint Maria Magdalene. The hospital was run by nuns who belonged to the Order of Hospitallers, and was also funded and built by the Amalfitans.[85] It seems that there were two separate hospitals, with the men tended by the Brothers and the women cared for by nursing sisters. According to Riley-Smith, the women's hospital was an independent institution which was not affiliated with the Hospitaller's institution,[86] despite the fact that both initially operated according to the Benedictine statutes and despite the geographical proximity between them.[87] In any event, the women's hospital was divided into wards and operated in a manner similar to that of the men's hospital.[88]

Medical staff and rules of ethics

The medical staff at the Hospitaller's House of the Sick included physicians, surgeons, blood-letters, pharmacists, and brothers. The physicians were supposed to have had the very finest medical training and were required to demonstrate the highest skill, reminiscent of modern medical techniques:

> "It is decreed by consent of the Brothers that for the benefit of the sick at the house of the sick in Jerusalem it is necessary that there be four physicians, who are qualified to examine urine, and to diagnose the different diseases and who are able to administer the appropriate medicines."[89]

[82] Nilsson & Sunzel, p. 19.
[83] Adington, Hospital, p. XVII.
[84] See: Felix Fabri, in: PPTS, VII-VIII, p. 395.
[85] Delaville, pp. 299-300; Riley-Smith, pp. 240-242; King, p. 12.
[86] Riley-Smith, p. 241, fn. 1.
[87] On the location of the women's hospital, see: Patrich, Structure, p. 12; King, p. 12.
[88] Adington, Hospital, p. XIV.
[89] Hospitaller documents, no. 627, p. 426.

The major function of the physicians concentrated on visiting the sick twice a day, morning and evening. At every visit, the physician checked the patient's pulse and urine. The physician was accompanied by two 'sergeants': one carried the basic medicines, such as syrups (sweetened with sugar); Oxymel (a potion made of honey and vinegar or sugar and vinegar, known in the Arab medical literature by the name of "sacanjebin"). The other sergeant carried the urine sample and after testing, ensured that it was discarded and the urinal cleaned. He also recorded the physician's dietary instructions.[90]

Assuming that the hospital accommodated some thousand people and employed four physicians according to the standard required, this means that every physician was responsible for two hundred and fifty patients. On the premise that each patient was examined for one minute, it appears that every doctor's round lasted over four hours, and this was done twice a day. This calculation would demonstrate that the job of a physician in public service for the Order was very arduous. The pressure must have increased at times when the number of patients grew or when there was a scarcity of physicians, and inevitably, the first to be effected were the patients who were receiving only minimal medical care to begin with. The high rate of mortality at the hospital (approximately fifty people died daily, according to John of Würzburg) proves that in spite of the impressive medical organization, which is similar to the modern standard, success in treating the sick was very low when compared with modern medical practice.

In addition, the physician was required to meet moral standards related to the rules of professional ethics. The physicians who were employed at the Hospitaller's House of the Sick were called upon to swear an "oath".[91] This was apparently the physicians' oath which was accepted either in the classical version attributed to Hippocrates (460-370 BCE) or in the Christian version.[92] We have no information about the identity of the physicians, their religion, or origins. It seems that the physicians were generally members of the Order. In fact the statutes of the Order make no mention of a brother-physician and it would therefore seem that they were private physicians, Franks or eastern Christians. These physicians received a salary for their services and were employed exclusively by the hospital.

In addition to the physicians, the hospital also employed surgeons and blood-letters (cuppers) who largely treated battle wounds; however, for regular procedures, the surgeons were generally considered professionally inferior in status to the physicians.[93] A document dated 1184 mentions that according to the standard, there were supposed to be four surgeons at the hospital.[94] There were also pharmacists at the hospital who prepared the potions and medications prescribed by the physicians.

---

[90] Adington, Hospital, p. XIII.
[91] Adington, Hospital, p. XV.
[92] Nilsson & Sunzel, pp. 17-18.
[93] Adington, Hospital, p. XIII-XIV.
[94] Hospitaller documents, no. 690, p. 458.

The hospital was divided into nine wards and according to one version, into eleven[95], but there is no evidence available that this classification was by types of disease and level of risk or classification of patients by age or different types of population.

Most of the work at the hospital was carried out by a large staff of brothers who were supposed to supervise and monitor the patients at all hours of the day and night. Every ward and section of the hospital was serviced by nine sergeants, to wit, knights of a low rank who constituted the major work force. Among their duties was washing the head and feet of the sick, changing the bed-sheets and making the beds, feeding them, and in effect, providing the weak patients with all of their needs.[96] Twice a week on hot days, the feet of the patients were washed and scrubbed with a pumice stone. One of the brothers was a barber who made sure that the heads and beards of the patients were tended. In order to improve the smell, incense was periodically used.[97] [Fig. 13]

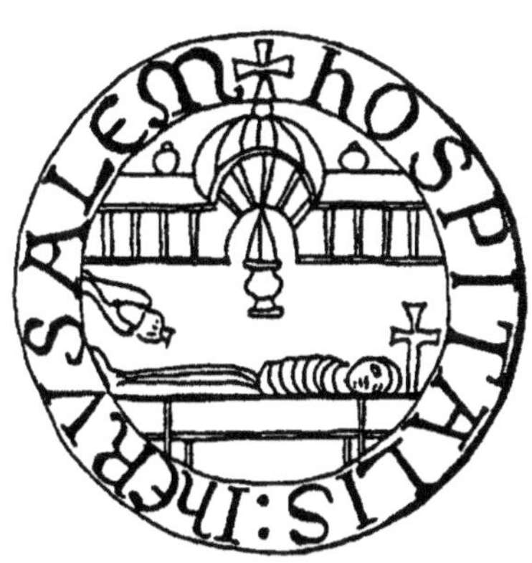

Figure 13: Seal of the Order of Hospitallers.

Another version of the statutes states that there must be twelve sergeants on every ward, and in addition, two nursing brothers and sixteen sergeants who supervised the patients at night in shifts. The sergeants were supposed to provide the patients with all their needs in a courteous manner, and this included: to put back their coverlets if they fell off the bed, to help them to the latrines, or if necessary to bring them bedpans and to empty them, to clean beds which had become soiled, and to change the linen sheets as needed.[98] One of the pilgrims who was given such treatment adds that the sergeants would also bring lamps to provide light for the patients who had to get dressed, would help them lie back comfortably, and when necessary, would bring a priest to administer the last sacraments to patients who had died and they later removed the bodies from the hospital.[99] The cemetery where the patients from the Hospitaller's House were buried was located in the site "Hakal Dama" outside the city walls, past the southeastern corner of the city.[100] The function of burying the dead also appears in the seal of the Order of Hospitallers which shows a building founded on pillars; in the center there is a cupola from which a lamp is suspended. The figure of dead person in a shroud is shown lying on a bed, with a cross at his head; opposite the cross is an upraised vessel, probably a censer.[101]

[95] Adington, Hospital, p. XI.
[96] Hospitaller documents, no. 627, p. 427.
[97] Adington, Hospital, p. XIV.
[98] Adington, Hospital, p. X-XI.
[99] Adington, Hospital, p. XIV.
[100] Ernoul, p.45; Hospitaller documents, no. 150, pp. 121-122.
[101] Prawer, Epigraphy, p. 386.

The ongoing treatment of the sick was an arduous and wearying job which must have effected the behavior and attitude of some of the brothers toward the sick. That is the reason that the Order's statutes repeatedly stress the directions to the masters and brothers of the Order to serve the sick gladly, devotedly, and uncomplainingly. In the event that one of the nursing brothers behaved rudely, in contravention of these directions, it was to be brought to the attention of the master of the Order who had to punish him in accordance with the statutes of the Order.[102]

A most interesting subject is the relationship between the statues of the Hospitaller's House of the Sick in Jerusalem and the "Assises of Jerusalem" whose writing was completed in the first half of the thirteenth century, circa 1240.[103] In the Assises of Jerusalem there are many sections (especially in chapter 236) that relate to the rules of medical ethics and the preservation of medical standards, legislation dealing with how licensing was granted to practice medicine, legislation against doctors who were not qualified, and the means of penalizing those doctors who harmed patients through negligence.[104]

One of the laws (chapter 238) stated that any foreign doctor who arrived from Christian Europe or lands under Muslim occupation was not permitted to practice medicine until he was tested by the best doctors in the country on his expertise in diagnosing by urine, in the presence of the bishop who gave his official permission. A doctor who did not pass the test and who did not receive a license from the bourgeois court was compelled to leave the city or pledge not to practice medicine.[105] There is dispute around the assumption that this legislation reflects the reality during the period of the First Crusade (until 1187).[106] There is no certainty that this legislation was actually enforced in the hospital run by the Hospitallers. More precisely, the instructions to test the doctor's skill and training (e.g. using the urine test) did exist but it is highly doubtful whether the law was enforced and whether the penalties were actually imposed on doctors who did not meet the medical standards. The legislation was not appropriate to the nature of the hospital in Jerusalem which treated the masses at no charge. The few physicians who worked at the hospital, even if they had wished, could not have given the kind of personal, devoted care to each of the patients which private medicine permits. In the final analysis, the hospital was a charitable institution designed to give refuge and lodging to the pilgrims and the poor, so that caring for the sick was only part of this service rather than its main purpose. Furthermore, the Assises of Jerusalem relate explicitly to the legal issue of a physician who treated slaves or freemen[107] rather than treating the sick within a public framework. It would seem that this legislation and the regulation of the medical profession were in practice in Jerusalem (until 1187), as part of private medical practice for the bourgeois and the nobility. Evidence of this may be found in a description of

---

[102] Hospitaller documents, no. 627, p. 426.
[103] Prawer, Institutions, p. 266.
[104] Wickeresheimer, pp. 694-696.
[105] Assises, p. 169. For a discussion of this legislation, see: Amundsen, pp. 517-522; Woodings, p. 269.
[106] Amundsen, pp. 517-520.
[107] Assises, chap. 236, p. 164-166.

the sickness of King Amalric I (1162-1174) who suffered from dysentery and fever. He summoned eastern physicians and demanded emphatically that they give him purgative drugs. They refused, apparently because they believed that what he was demanding would only do him further harm rather than cure him. Left with no other choice, he summoned Frankish doctors and presented his demand, adding that he did not care what the result would be, and that he bore responsibility for the outcome, and they agreed.[108] This shows that there was a system of legislative deterrence against doctors who practiced medicine in way that was considered unreasonable and flew in the face of accepted practice; in such a case they might have paid a penalty, even with their lives. It is interesting that according to this story, the eastern physicians are presented as skilled doctors with a high level of ethics, corresponding to the rules of medical ethics that obligated them, while the Franks are depicted as physicians who contravened the medical standards.

Statues of the Order: Actual versus ideal

Most of the information that we have cited about the functioning of the Knights' hospital is derived from the statutes and directives that were decided upon in the conferences of the Order which wished to chart a general, ideal framework for the proper functioning of the hospital. However, it appears that things did not always run according to the directives in terms of: the number of physicians and level of training, the organization of manpower, and the provision of food and equipment to the patients. In contrast, descriptions of the visitors who came to the hospital reflect a more realistic situation. The comparison between the travelers' descriptions and the statutes shows that usually there was not a great discrepancy between the ideal and the actual, particularly during the period that the Order flourished economically. The directives laid down by the Order were ultimately carried out depending on the resources and the manpower available at any given period.

Financing the hospital's expenses

The managing of such a large institution required an operating budget to maintain the building, furniture, food, and medicine. Thus, for example, to pay for hiring the services of the doctors and to buy almonds for the patients, a sum of 1500 byzantimes was required.[109] The source of funding came from contributions and gifts and from the profits of the extensive properties owned by the Order in Europe and controlled by the Crusader Kingdom of Jerusalem.[110] In Hospitaller documents there are references to dozens of villages and estates in Judea, Samaria, and the coastal plain which had been purchased or conferred as a gift upon the St. John's Hospital in Jerusalem.[111] Every year one third of the revenues collected by the Hospitallers in Europe

[108] William of Tyre, XX, 31.
[109] Adington, Hospital, p. X.
[110] Prawer, Colonial, p. 340.
[111] E.g., Hospitaller documents, no. 115, p. 97; no. 116, pp. 97-98; no. 621, pp. 421-422.

were sent to the main branch in the land of Israel.[112] The branches of the Order in France, in the Italian cities, Antioch, and throughout the Kingdom of Jerusalem sent equipment or its equivalent, depending on the decisions of the heads of the Order. The equipment included cloth and cotton for sheets and blankets and a supply of sugar for medicines. An illustrative example may be seen in one of the decisions made by the general meeting of the Hospitallers on 14.3.1182:

"It was also decreed when the council [Chapter-General] of the brethren was held, that the Prior of the Hospital of France should send each year to Jerusalem one hundred sheets of dyed cotton (*dras de coton tainz*) to replace the coverlets of the sick poor... The Prior of Italy each year should send to Jerusalem for our lords the sick two thousand ells of fustian [coarse twilled cotton fabric] of divers colors...and the Prior of Pisa should send likewise the like number of fustians. And the Prior of Venice likewise... And likewise the Bailiffs this side of sea ...of whom the Bailiff of Antioch should send to Jerusalem two thousand ells of cotton cloth for the coverlets of the poor. The Prior of Mont Pelerin [i.e. Tripoli] should send to Jerusalem two quintals (i.e. 200 pounds) of sugar for the syrups, and the medicines and the electuaries [medicinal powders made up with honey or sugar] of the sick. For this same service the Bailiff of Tabarie (Tiberias) should send them the same quantity. The Prior of Constantinople should send for the sick two hundred felts...[113]

The Order of Teutonic Knights

The Order of Teutonic Knights was established to provide services to the German-speaking pilgrims, the poor and the sick. It began as a private initiative funded by a Teutonic couple who settled in the city and it subsequently turned into an order of German knights.[114] First created in the first half of the twelfth century as an appendage of the Hospitallers,[115] the center of the Teutonic Order was the Church of St. Maria in Jerusalem in a location known in recent generations as the Jewish Quarter of Jerusalem's Old City. Members of the German organization wished their order to be independent but official recognition of the order only came after the Third Crusade (1190). In any event, while still affiliated with the Order of the Hospitallers they won their autonomy which enabled them at that stage to establish a smaller hospital in Jerusalem which functioned in the same format as the Knights' Hospital. [116]

[112] Riley-Smith, p. 340.
[113] Hospitaller documents, no. 627, pp. 426-427.
[114] According to Jacques de Vitry; see: PPTS, XI, p. 55.
[115] Felix Fabri at the end of the fifteenth century mentions the remnants of the Teuton hostel near the St. John's Hospital in: PPTS, VII-VIII, p. 395.
[116] Prawer, Colonial, pp. 347-352.

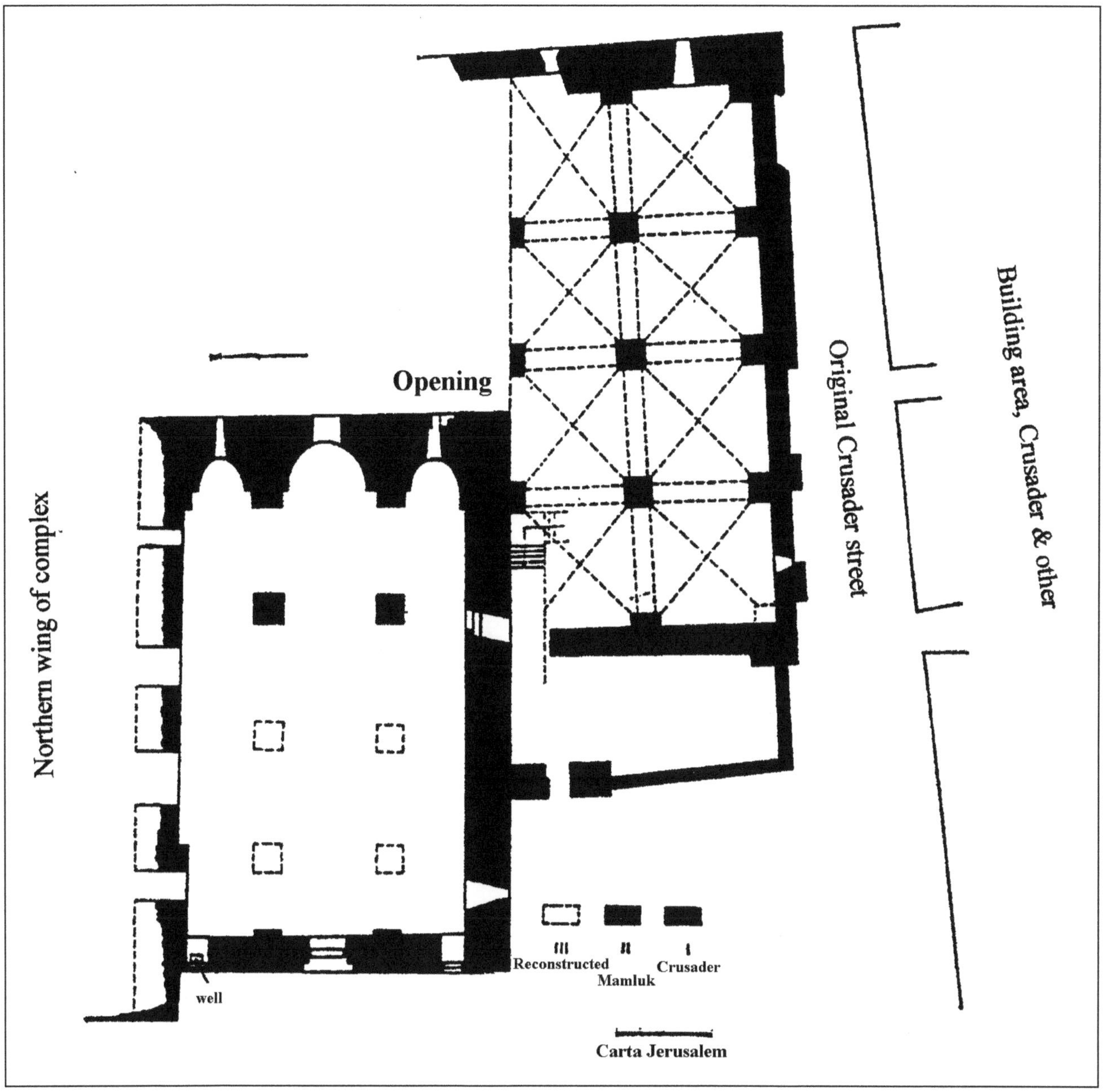

Figure 14: Plan of the Crusader Church complex where the Germanic hospital was apparently situated.

Documents from the archives of the Teutonic Knights from 1173 and 1177 mention the sugar produced for the sick in the city of Shechem (Nablus), which the Teutonic Order would receive every year from the farmers as an agricultural tax.[117] However, it may be that these are forged documents which should be attributed to a period later than 1220.[118] Archaeological excavations carried out on the site uncovered a Crusader church. The excavators believe that the complex of buildings adjacent to it should be associated

[117] Strehlke, p. 7, no. 6; p. 9, no. 8.

[118] Prawer, Colonial, p. 351, fn. 37. The document from 1177 attributed to King Amalric is problematic since he died three years earlier.

with the Germanic hospital. [Fig. 14] This building was apparently destroyed when Jerusalem was conquered by Saladin (1187).[119]

The Order of Lepers (St. Lazarus)

Another organization that was involved in providing medical care in Jerusalem was the Order of Leprous Knights named in honor of St. Lazarus (Luke 16:20).[120] This order was founded in the first half of the twelfth century and in time, turned into a military order as well. In a document dated 1147 there is explicit reference to "the leprous brethren in Jerusalem".[121] The center of the order was the "Domus Leprosorum" which lay beyond the northern wall of the city of Jerusalem, near what is known today as "the New Gate". [122] In this area, whose precise location is still not clear, was the "Wicket of St. Lazarus" which was the exit from the city to the lepers' hospital.[123] The exact location of the leprosarium has not been identified conclusively. The archaeological excavations conducted there while preparing the ground for a new building for the Jerusalem municipality uncovered a large public building, where the technique of stonecutting employed must be dated to the Crusader Period. Based on the dating and location of the building as compared with documentation from that period, the archaeologists raised the hypothesis that this was the leprosarium.[124] The Church of St. Lazarus, and the leprosarium also appear in medieval maps of Jerusalem.[125]

The main purpose of this order was to treat lepers, considered in the Middle Ages to be incurable and ostracized by society. In this way it provided a fine humanitarian service on the one hand while isolating the lepers from society on the other. We have no information about the manner in which the order was organized and the medical techniques it employed but it is fair to assume that that it was influenced by the organizational methods of the other orders, adapting them to its own special needs. Besides the knights, there were also lay brothers who served in the order, as well as ten slaves, this according to a document from Jerusalem in 1164.[126]

This order received official recognition and independence, which was reflected in the seal of the Order. The seal shows the figure of a leper, his face ravaged by illness, his head enveloped in a cap. One hand is partially hidden (perhaps also afflicted) and the other is holding a noise-maker, which was used to warn the public of his approach [Fig. 15]. Like the other orders, this one also had properties and branches in the city of Jerusalem and other regions of the country. Thanks to the privileges, donations, and properties it owned,

[119] Ovadiah, Church, p. 212.
[120] Wickeresheimer, pp. 700-701.
[121] Lazare documents, no. 4, p. 125.
[122] Prawer, Colonial, p. 354.
[123] Bahat, Topography, pp. 27, 74.
[124] Report of D. Bahat and A. Maeir in: Kroyanker, pp. 324-325.
[125] Levy, Maps, pp. 429, 476.
[126] Lazare documents, no. 22, p. 140.

the Order could finance the operating of the hospital. The first privilege mentioned in the documents was granted by the patriarch of Jerusalem between 1130-1145.[127] Among the Order's many properties was the mill close to David's Gate. Later this was destroyed by instruction of Queen Melisenda (1151) and in exchange, the Order was awarded a vineyard near Bethlehem.[128] From documents of the Order of Lepers, it appears that it continued to engage in healing the sick during the Ayyubid Period as well. In a document from 1234, the reign of Frederich II in Jerusalem, we hear of many properties near Caesaria being granted to the Grandmaster of the Order of Lepers in Jerusalem.[129]

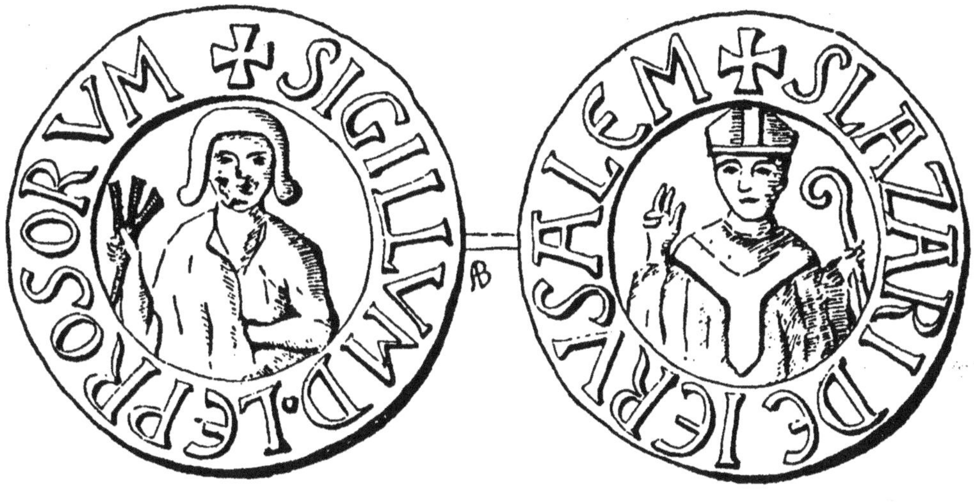

Figure 15: Seal of the Order of Lazarus.

It is of special interest to consider the social status and depiction of the leper in the Kingdom of Jerusalem. As opposed to what was accepted in Europe, the lepers of the Order of St. Lazarus succeeded in taking an active role in the life of the Kingdom and the defense of its borders. In Europe, people of all classes (citizens, nobility, and clergy) who were afflicted with leprosy were forced to leave their positions.[130] The Order of St. Lazarus which was initially founded for indigent lepers also provided a respectable solution for brothers who fell ill. Members of the order of lepers were active partners in managing the institution and were even headed by a master who was himself a leper. The afflicted knights continued to fulfill their functions as fighters alongside the healthy knights. Their rights were also safeguarded when it came to personal status: they continued to benefit from their estates and revenues and could bequeath their wealth to whomever they wished.[131]

---

[127] Lazare documents, no. 1, p. 123.

[128] Lazare documents, no. 10, p. 130. For more on the Order's property in Jerusalem and environs, see documents: nos. 2-3, 5, 11, 16.

[129] Lazare documents, no. 37, p. 154; no. 38, pp. 154-155.

[130] Shahar, Lepers, pp. 22-24.

[131] Shahar, Lepers, pp. 25-31; Viztum, pp. 39-40.

The change in image of the leper in Crusader society was undoubtedly the result of the establishment of the center in Jerusalem and of an understanding of the leper's needs by the Frankish policy makers. The explanation for the special status the lepers were accorded in the Crusader Kingdom is also related to the fact that some of the royalty themselves fell victim to the disease, such as the daughter of King Polak.[132] It is of especial note that the king who headed the crusader Kingdom of Jerusalem for several years was Baldwin IV (1174-1185) who was afflicted with leprosy. Despite his severe illness and his youthful age, he succeeded in guiding the kingdom judiciously.[133] This extraordinary phenomenon of lepers in the Kingdom of Jerusalem may also be explained against the background of a constant shortage of fighting soldiers. The lepers, in the first stage of the disease, were physically fit and could be put to use. And indeed, this order did supply faithful manpower endowed with high motivation and military ability.[134] Thus for example, we know that lepers, along with the other military orders, took part in the Battle of Herbeya (near Gaza) in 1244, where many met their death.[135]

The Crusaders and Muslim medicine

There are many opinions among scholars regarding the extent of involvement by the Franks in the life and settlement of the land of Israel. This issue is connected with the more complex question of the relationship between Crusader medicine and eastern medicine. To phrase it differently, what was the standard of Frankish medicine as compared with the local, eastern medicine, and what medical techniques did the Crusaders usually prefer to use? We cannot discuss the entire complex of issues here, and we will therefore treat the narrow aspect of the history of medicine in Jerusalem. There is scant material about the standard of Frankish physicians in the Kingdom of Jerusalem. Best known are the descriptions of Usama Ibn Munqid (1095-1188) who portrays the Frankish physicians in a negative and ludicrous manner, depicting them as ignoramuses who hold superstitious beliefs, lacking even the most fundamental knowledge of modern medical practice as compared with the eastern physicians.[136] Although this is an exaggerated and tendentious description, one may assume that eastern medicine was far superior to Frankish medicine. Adington who discusses Crusader medical knowledge in the first generation of their conquest, notes the absence of magical-religion in the healing process, a phenomenon which had been quite widespread in western medicine at that time. The Franks held a practical approach to matters in the land of Israel was practical, and this explains how the Crusaders could learn from western medicine and adopt its principles without psychological or practical reservation.[137] In contrast, Conrad contends that there must be a re-examination of the descriptions given by Usama Ibn Munqid and the other sources dealing with the relationship between Frankish medicine and

[132] Fort, p. 333.
[133] William of Tyre, XXII, 25; Shahar, Lepers, pp. 37-38.
[134] Shahar, Groups, p. 80.
[135] Prawer, Kingdom, II, p. 300.
[136] Ibn Munqid, pp. 132-134; Woodings, pp. 270-271.
[137] Adington, Knowledge, pp. 320-326.

eastern medicine in the period of the Crusader Kingdom of Jerusalem, and he challenges the accepted premise that western medicine was inferior.[138]

The documentation that refers to private medical treatment in Jerusalem or medicine provided through the various orders of knights does not usually mention who the physicians were. We have only two examples where there is actual mention of the origins of the physicians, and both indicate that the Frankish rulers preferred to employ the services of the eastern physicians.

The first example is that of the physician Abu Suliman Daud b.Abi al-Mani b. Abi Fana who was brought by the Crusader King Amalric to Jerusalem with his entire family.[139] An account is told of that same king that when he fell sick, he preferred to first call for eastern physicians ("Greeks, Syrians, and other nations who were well-known for their expertise in disease") and only afterwards did he summon Frankish doctors.[140] There is another indirect description connected to a Christian physician, a native of Jerusalem named Yaqub Ibn Siqlab. A year after the Battle of the Horns of Hattin he went to Damascus for further training and to practice medicine with the personal physician of Saladin, first clothed in blue attire in the manner of the Frankish physicians.[141] This account attests to the fact that the eastern doctors in Jerusalem adopted the Frankish mode of dress, and it may even imply that Y'aqub Ibn Siqlab first worked for Franks of the higher classes even before he offered his services to the Ayyubs who conquered Jerusalem.

One may assume that at least in some of the cases where there are casual references to doctors who tended the Crusader leaders of Jerusalem, this refers to physicians of Eastern Christian origin. As we have seen in the period preceding the Crusader conquest, the medical profession in Jerusalem was well-developed and the tendency to favor eastern physicians over Frankish physicians was apparently widespread.[142] This is reflected in the words of William of Tyre, chronicler of the Crusader Period, who finds it hard to accept this phenomenon:

> "...for our Eastern princes, through the influence of their women, scorn the medicines and practice of our Latin physicians and believe only in the Jews, Samaritans, Syrians, and Saracens. Most recklessly they put themselves under the care of such practitioners and trust their lives to people who are ignorant of the science of medicine."[143]

---

[138] Conrad, pp. XXVII- LII.
[139] Ibn abi Usaybi'a, pp. 587-589.
[140] William of Tyre, XX, 31.
[141] Ibn abi Usaybi'a, p. 654.
[142] See: Amundsen, p. 521, fn. 16.
[143] William of Tyre, XVIII, 34.

This also is evidence of the assimilation of the Crusaders in the land of Israel and its culture. Thus for example, we know that most of the kings of Jerusalem married non-Latin wives, among them Baldwin I, II, and III, and Amalric I. These queens, with the encouragement of their husbands, promoted the interests of the local Christians and helped in the preservation of their customs.[144]

The professional literature contains copious reference to the subject of the level of medical knowledge possessed by the Franks and the extent to which they were influenced by Eastern medicine. In the course of research several examples were brought of methods of healing, medical standards, and the organization of a medical institution that were accepted practice in the Jerusalem region, such as: diagnoses made using urine, treatment using cautery and scalding, rules of medical ethics and the treatment of the patient, the physician's oath, licensed medicine, supervision, and penal laws for physicians accused of malpractice, the operation of hospitals and organization by medical wards, etc. For each of these examples,one may bring proof that they were known at that time both in the East as well as in the West, and it would be superfluous to elaborate here. It is important to mention that is not always possible to precisely follow the spread and transfer of these medical techniques in the encounter between European culture and the areas under Muslim rule. While the settlement of Franks in the Kingdom of Jerusalem and their encounter with the local culture may be an adequate explanation, it appears to be only superficially satisfactory. One must recall that ultimately, medical technique, Frankish as well as Arab, was founded on a common basis, namely, the school of classical medicine. Therefore the Franks did not find it difficult to accept eastern medicine and to adhere to it. Furthermore, mutual influences were at work at additional points of contact, such as at Salerno in southern Italy or in Sicily during the time of Roger I and Roger II (1130-1154).[145]

---

[144] Miller, Knights, p. 727; Rose, p. 176.
[145] See further Conrad's article, pp. XLII-XLIII.

Summary:

The information on medical services in Jerusalem during the Crusader period is fragmentary and presents only a partial picture which was more representative of the elite ruling class in Frankish society. The sources show that during the period of the First Kingdom there were several frameworks in Jerusalem and the environs that were capable of providing medical services. The first framework was that of the Eastern Christians, and that was based on knowledge and trained personnel from the monastic movement of the Judean Desert. The second was that provided by Eastern Christian and Latin physicians who practiced medicine in the private sector on the basis of supply and demand, and this was apparently under supervision like nearly everything else in the kingdom. The Eastern Christian physicians seem to have also provided medical services to the rural Muslim population around Jerusalem (in the city proper, there were no Muslims). Some of the Eastern Christian doctors were employed by the bourgeois and the Frankish aristocracy. In addition to these were the Frankish physicians about whom little information is available.

Most of the information at hand relates to the system of medical services provided by the military orders, and in particular, the St. John's Hospital of the Knights of the Hospitaller Order, which provided medical services to the pilgrims and the poor. The establishment of hospitals and institutions of philanthropy was a familiar phenomenon in both the East and the West but from the European point of view, one may point to two innovations in the Jerusalem type of institution. The first was in establishing a large, sophisticated hospital that was capable of accommodating hundreds of people at once, by setting up an organizational and economic infrastructure that was able to carry out sustained activity over time. The innovative quality was also reflected in the very existence of a "real" hospital, that functioned as a medical institution par excellence. It is possible that the Knights Hospital in Jerusalem served as a successful examplar and prototype that brought about the establishment of hospitals on similar lines in Europe.[146] It is almost indisputable that hospitals in a format similar to that of the Hospitallers' also existed in the Near East, and as we have seen in Jerusalem proper during the Byzantine and Early Muslim periods. In example, we can note Rabbi Benjamin of Tudela who describes with wonder the Muslim hospital in Baghdad;[147] in contrast, his description of the hospital in Jerusalem is more reserved.[148] One must not forget that in the final analysis the hospital in Jerusalem was not established by the Hospitallers; it had been built many years earlier before the Crusader conquest, under Muslim rule, at a time when it was Eastern Christians who were preeminent in the medical sciences. Thus all the indications are that the source of inspiration for the establishment of the hospital by the Hospitallers was either Byzantine or Muslim,[149] and the novelty was in that it was adopted by the Franks.

[146] Miller, Knights, p. 733; Dolev, p. 137.
[147] Adler, pp. 37-38.
[148] Seide, pp. 403-404.
[149] Miller, Knights, pp. 723-733; Riley-Smith, p. 335.

The second innovation of the military orders was the concept that medical care was given by warrior knights who considered it a supreme ideal. Practically speaking, the orders continued the traditional role that Byzantine monasticism had undertaken at its inception. Beyond the humanitarian aspect, the purpose was to encourage and sustain the pilgrim movement which was both an ideological as well as economic corridor between western Europe and the Holy Land, with its center in Jerusalem.

An examination of the activity of the Crusader orders of knights shows that the crowning glory of their activity in terms of medicine was indisputably the Knights' Hospital in Jerusalem. This institution reached its climax of development and activity in the seventies and eighties of the twelfth century. The scope of its activity certainly grew as a result of the increase in battle casualties with the Muslims who threatened the Kingdom of Jerusalem. The conquest of Jerusalem by Saladin in 1187 led to a halt in the activity of this institution (except for a short period of time) and began a new era in the history of medicine in Jerusalem.

Chapter Five

The Ayyubid Period (1187-1250)

Introduction

With his conquest of Jerusalem in 1187, Saladin imparted to the city its Muslim hallmarks and characteristics. He tried to blur the impressions left by the Crusaders and to mark the city with his own distinctive imprint. The Franks were forced to leave Jerusalem while the Eastern Christians remained firmly in place. Saladin encouraged both Moslems and Jews to settle in the city, and that marks a turning point in the demographic and social character of the city. All of these changes also had important effects on the status of medicine in Jerusalem.

However, a discussion of medicine in Jerusalem during the Ayyubid period must be prefaced by an examination of the changes that had taken place in this field throughout the region at that time, in Syria and the Land of Israel (al-Sham). The science of medicine, which was of such importance throughout the Near East all through the medieval period, made impressive achievements during the Ayyubid Period, particularly during the rule of Saladin (1174-1193) and his heirs. During a major part of the Ayyubid period, the administrative center moved to Damascus, which had a strong influence on the development of medicine in Greater Syria by virtue of its becoming an important medical center. The Ayyubid rulers ordered many hospitals built all over the Near East, particularly in Syria,[1] and with their encouragement, renowned physicians were invited to serve there, as well as to serve the populace of the royal court. The building of hospitals and institutions of philanthropy as well as the institution of the court physician were already familiar and well-developed from the time of Nur al-Din, but during the rule of Saladin these developments reached heights which had never previously been documented. Every ruler had several physicians of differing ranks; some were personal physicians who received a fixed salary while others were summoned as needed. Ministers and lesser officials in the administration retained their own physicians, a practice which bespoke an elevated social status.[2] According to Ibn Abi Usaybi'a in his survey essay, Saladin was served by no fewer than twenty-one physicians: eight Muslims, eight Jews, and five Christians.[3] Seven of the physicians were in Egypt and eleven in Syria.[4]

Most of the information on physicians of that period is based on two writers who wrote essays dedicated to the history of physicians until their own times. The first was Ibn al-Qifti (1171-1248) and the second was Ibn Abi Usaybi'a (1203-1270). Both writers belonged to families close to the inner circles of the Ayyubid rule

---

[1] Hamarneh, Development, pp. 371-373.
[2] Jadon, Physicians, pp. 323-340; Edde, pp. 91-109.
[3] See: Meyerhof, p. 169.
[4] Jadon, Comparison, p. 65.

who were active in the region consisting of Syria, the Land of Israel, and Egypt. It would seem that the appearance of these essays precisely during that period is not coincidental and reflects the prominent status of medicine, at least among the ruling class. The information that they bring describes only the prominent physicians and does not refer to the numerous other doctors who were active at that time throughout Syria and particularly in Jerusalem.

The medical sciences in al-Sham became a thriving and highly developed industry during the Ayyubid period.[5] The study and practice of medicine made wide inroads even among those strata of the population who were not members of the profession. The proliferation of medical treatises written at the time constitutes an additional gauge for reconstructing the extent to which medicine flourished and how thoroughly medical services reached the various strata of society. Most of these essays were written for the rulers or at their behest, and it appears that it must have been easier for physicians of means and connections to devote their time to writing books and ensuring their dissemination. In example, one may point out that nearly half of Saladin's doctors wrote medical books.[6] This reality must have transformed al-Sham into a center of medical scholarship which attracted learned practitioners from even more remote places.[7]

All of the activities mentioned here leave a positive impression regarding the enhanced status of medicine in al-Sham during the Ayyubid period. At the same time it should be noted that for the people of that era, this was, paradoxically, a period of decline in the status of medicine. The information available indicates that Saladin as well as the preeminent physicians of his times such as al-Baghdadi were not satisfied with the level of doctors they encountered.[8] Saladin discussed the professional standards of the physicians in Damascus with the Jewish physician Ibn Jumay' and following this discussion, the latter wrote an article entitled: "Treatise to Saladin on the Revival of the Art of Medicine".

According to Ibn Jumay', the major reasons for the decline in medicine was an inadequate knowledge of the science of anatomy, the failure to devote oneself to this science as required by the school of Galenus, and the abandoning of study from the original writings of Hippocrates and Galenus by translating them into Arabic. In order to improve the professional standards of physicians, he recommended intensive study of the fundamental textbooks of classical medicine, that medical students must get practical training in hospitals and physicians must be tested before they practice medicine, and their work must be under supervision.[9] It

[5] Klein-Franke, p. 105.

[6] Jadon, Comparison, p. 70; five out of the fifteen physicians in Syria and four out of the seven physicians in Egypt.

[7] On the phenomenon of the migration of physicians to al-Sham from various regions around the world, see: Murad, pp. 228-231; Edde, p. 94.

[8] There is no doubt that the development of the medical system in the Ayyubid Period and transforming it into a commodity available to all also led to the thriving of untrained doctors and great competition and disputes between them. These things may be learned from the writings of Maimonides who came out against the widespread phenomenon in Egypt among "both the great and the common" to travel from one physician to another in order to obtain medical treatment,. See: Maimonides, Asthma, pp. 117-118.

[9] The first review of a treatise by Ibn Jumay' was given by Meyerhof, Physician, pp. 169-178. The treatise was published by Fandrich and a summary may be found in Jadon, Comparison, pp. 74-75.

may be that Ibn Jumay' was right and that at that time the status of medicine was ignoble as compared to a previous age (the ninth and tenth centuries), though this is not the place to examine the point. However, his criticism may also attest to the heightened awareness and importance that Saladin ascribed to the medical sciences and his willingness to improve the situation.

Medicine in Jerusalem: Between the Franks and the Ayyubs

The centrality of Jerusalem in the Muslim world, which led to the development of medicine in the city, was to a large extent a result of the singular policy pursued by Saladin, founder of the Ayyubid dynasty. After his death,[10] the city again began to decline due to disputes and struggles among his many heirs. One of the results of these schisms which began in the Ayubid camp was the Tel-'Ajul – Jaffa agreement wherein Jerusalem was transferred (1229) to Crusader rule for approximately 15 years. Thus, any discussion of the status of medicine in Jerusalem in the Ayyubid period is primarily connected with the period of Saladin's rule over the city (1187-1193). Saladin must be credited with the establishment of the city's Muslim hospital and encouraging physicians to settle there, as well as additional initiatives. There is a wealth of information on activity in the field of medicine after his death, but even at best, only about the continuity in policy charted by Saladin in all matters related to the public and governmental health system.

The distinction that we seem to be drawing here regarding the history of medicine in Jerusalem between the Crusader Period and the Ayyubid is somewhat artificial. In the previous chapter, it was demonstrated that the Franks were influenced to a certain extent during the period of the First Kingdom by local medicine as far as medical treatment, the use of materia medica, and the use of Eastern physicians. It would appear that the physicians were the major mediating factor between the Franks and the Muslims. From both the medical aspect, as well as commercial considerations, we know that it was possible to transfer people and merchandise between the two rival powers despite the tension and hostility between them.[11] It may be that physicians were considered a neutral factor due to their profession of saving human lives no matter whose they were, and apparently there were doctors who supplied services to the Muslims and Franks alike. It is clearer that there were physicians who had worked for the Franks and with the transfer of rule, were readily welcomed by the Ayyubids. The physicians who were under the protection of the realm (Jews and Christians) were accorded a status identical to that accorded the Muslim physicians.[12]

For the purpose of illustration, let us consider two examples. The first is the story of the Egyptian physician Abu Suliman Daud ibn al-Mani ibn Abi Fana. who was brought to Jerusalem by the Crusader king Amalric I

[10] The Muslim chroniclers described in detail the progressive stages of Saladin's disease and how he was treated by the physicians up until his death, see: Ibn al- Attir al-Kamil, XII, pp. 39-40; Gabrieli, pp. 246-251.
[11] Ibn Jubayr, pp. 287-288; 298.
[12] Edde, pp. 91-93.

(ruled 1162-1174). Abu Suliman converted to Christianity and faithfully served the Frankish king, but this did not stop him from sending a message to Saladin with his son, a Crusader knight (!), telling him that he foretold in the stars that the king was destined to conquer Jerusalem. Saladin did not forget this, and after the conquest of Jerusalem, he showed kindness to the physician, granting him special status. Saladin paid him a handsome salary, and after Abu Suliman's death, ensured his children's future. Abu Suliman's son, the physician Ibn Sa'ed, never forget his Muslim heritage and intervened with the Frankish king on behalf of a prominent Muslim religious leader who was languishing in a Crusader prison, eventually bringing about his release.[13]

Another example is the case of the Christian physician Muwaffaq al-Din Ya'qub Siqab who apparently worked in the service of the Franks and then in the service of the Ayyubids. One of his sons, Sadid al-Din Abu Mansur, was a physician who converted to Islam[14] while his second son, the physician Rashid al-Din Abu Sa'ed, remained a Christian.[15] It would seem that for the physicians, religion was generally a matter of convenience with the objective of securing some of the privileges of power.[16]

Especially worthy of mention is the organization of the hospital as an institution, which without doubt received an impetus for development and progress under the Muslims and the Crusaders at the same time. Thus, for example, a description of the St. John's Hospital with the format of the new hospital established by Nur-al-Din in Damascus (completed in 1156) by Ibn Jubayr who visited the Holy Land in 1184 just before the Battle of the Horns of Hattin points out the many similarities between the two.[17] It would therefore seem that there were dimorphic influences between the Muslims and Franks and to a certain extent, the contact and encounters between these two forces contributed to this. It is hard to know what were the central factors that contributed to the development of the institution of the hospital, and it may be connected to the circumstances that prevailed at that time as a result of the spread of epidemics and disease[18], or perhaps the many wars between the Muslims and the Crusaders which demanded appropriate medical solutions for the thousands of wounded on both sides.[19] The exigencies of that time may be deduced from the fact that Nur al-Din ordered the building of hospitals with the ransom money paid by the Crusaders.[20] This joined the

[13] Ibn abi Usaybi'a, pp. 587-589.
[14] Ibn abi Usaybi'a, pp. 654, 699.
[15] Ibn abi Usaybi'a, pp. 599-600.
[16] There is also a famous story about Maimonides who was summoned to treat Richard the Lionhearted, King of England, and according to other versions, the king offered to make him his personal physician, but Maimonides declined. Bernard Lewis proved that this was apparently an apocryphal tale, see: Lewis, pp. 70-75.
[17] Ibn Jubayr, p. 283.
[18] Carstans, p. 670.
[19] Hamarneh, Development, p. 371; Jadon, Physicians, pp. 325-326.
[20] Sibt ibn al-Jawzi, p. 248; al-Dawadari, VII, p. 33.

strong awareness and vast knowledge he had on the subject of medicine[21] and his sympathy for men of science and religion which undoubtedly influenced Saladin.[22]

The military needs seem also to have been an important motivation in the development of medicine by Saladin. A hint of this may be found in a Muslim document which refers to Hassam al-Din 'Isa al-Jaraihi, an amir of the ruler Saladin for whom Zawiyat al-Jaraihiya in northern Jerusalem was named.[23] The nickname 'Jarah' attests to the person's profession and it means 'surgeon'; he may have treated the battle wounded and in gratitude for his service, was awarded an estate which was named after him.[24] Thus, when we consider the development of medicine after the Battle of the Horns of Hattin (1187), it is reasonable that the major factor operating here was the policy and personal involvement of Saladin. Echoes of this may be detected in the words of 'Abd al-Latif al-Baghdadi (1162-1231), one of the preeminent Muslim physicians who met Saladin in Jerusalem in 1191:

> "It was known that Saladin made a cease-fire treaty with the Crusaders and returned to Jerusalem, and I felt the need to appeal to him; accordingly, I took the books of the ancients which I was able to take and I set my face towards Jerusalem. I saw a great king who inspired wonder and love in the hearts of both near and far... the first night I was with him, I found an assemblage of men of science, who were discussing among themselves the fields of science, and he was most attentive and participated greatly. He began to speak about the way to build the walls and to dig the channels, and they agreed with him regarding these, and all that he said was wondrous. He was interested in building the wall of Jerusalem and digging its channel... Saladin gave me thirty dinars every month for the mosque office, and his children also gave me wages so that my monthly wage was one hundred dinars..."[25]

From this excerpt one may see, at least as the Muslim chroniclers presented it, the strong attachment Saladin had to Jerusalem on the one hand, and the way he cultivated scientific study on the other. Although Saladin was engaged in the fortification of Jerusalem for fear of a possible attack by the Franks, he also found the time to engage in scientific study. He established a council of scholars in Jerusalem and was an active participant in it, as the first among his peers. In order to encourage prominent theoreticians and scholars to settle in Jerusalem, he gave them incentives, offering them money and high status. The policy charted by Saladin was adopted by his heirs as well. One might then sum up by mentioning several areas where Saladin contributed to developing medicine in Jerusalem and turning the city into an important center among the centers of medicine in the Near East: building hospitals, encouraging physicians of other nationalities to

[21] An example of this is provided in a description of Nur al-Din's final hours, when he lay mortally ill surrounded by the finest doctors. When they examined him and wished to bleed him, he refused, saying that it was not accepted practice to bleed a man of sixty. See: Ibn al-Attir al-Kamil, XI, p. 403.

[22] See: Ibn al-Attir al-Kamil, XI, p. 405.

[23] Mujir al-Din, II, p. 48.

[24] The lands of Sheikh Jarah and the Waqf of Abu-Tor, both of whom were generals of Saladin, are mentioned, for example, in documents from the sixteenth century. See: Cohen, Jews, p. 224.

[25] Ibn abi Usaybi'a, p. 688.

settle there,[26] developing the institution of the royal court physicians, improving the professional standards of the physicians, and writing medical literature. Some of these will be discussed later on in more detail.

The hospital

One of the many activities carried out by Saladin in Jerusalem after it was conquered was the establishment of a hospital which is referred to in the sources as "al-Bimaristan al-Salahi". According to one of the chronicles, Saladin came to Jerusalem "and established it on a firm basis and designated the church that was on the street of the Holy Sepulchre as a hospital and sent to it healing drugs and medicines."[27]

Although this institution was considered one of Saladin's most renowned projects in Jerusalem, information about how it functioned is sparse and ambiguous. It is not clear whether it functioned on the format and scale of the Hospital of the Knights of St. John and whether it redefined its intended public or changed ownership.

From the Ayyubid Period we have two pieces of information that explicitly mention the activity of the hospital in Jerusalem and the physicians who served in it. The first item relates to Rashid al-Din al-Suri (1178-1242) who lived in Jerusalem for two years, and reportedly engaged in the practice of medicine in the hospital in that city.[28] The second piece of information relates to Muwaffaq al-Din Ya'qub ibn Siqlab, a local Christian physician who also worked at the public hospital until the Ayyubid ruler al-Malik al-Mu'azzam 'Isa took him along with him to Damascus (1219).[29] It is noteworthy that the reference to the hospital in both places is casual; it is not referred to as Saladin's hospital. It is not clear whether it is referring to another public hospital, of the like known in Jerusalem still from the First Muslim Period[30] or whether a new building had been built.[31]

This discussion is connected to the question of the populace that the al-Salahi Hospital was intended to serve. If we grant that Saladin only wished to change the ownership of the Frankish hospital and not its purpose, then the hospital was supposed to provide medical service only to the poor and the pilgrims, as the Hospitaller institution had operated. This idea conforms to the other philanthropic projects associated with it. This premise may reinforce the hypothesis that there was another hospital in Jerusalem that was designated for the other residents of the city.

[26] Klein-Franke, pp. 105, 125.
[27] Al-'Asali, Ma'ahid, p. 294, according to Nuwayri (the events of 1192).
[28] Ibn abi Usaybi'a, p. 700.
[29] Ibn al-Qifti, pp. 378-379.
[30] Khusraw, p. 21.
[31] See: Klein-Franke, pp. 121-122.

According to Mujir-al-Din one may definitely state that the al-Bimaristan al-Salahi was located near the spice market ("Attarin") on Dargah Street near the Church of the Holy Sepulcher.[32] In another place Mujir al-Din comments that in proximity to the al-Salahi Hospital stood Zawiyat al-Dargah in a building where the Hospital of the Knights of St. John was located during the time of the Franks, where a partially ruined minaret stood. [33] This shows that the al-Salahi hospital did not entirely take the place of the Frankish hospital or alternately, that it was merely located alongside it.

The latter assumption seems more reasonable. Explicit information is brought by the chronicler 'Imad al-Din according to which Saladin located the hospital at the church close to the Hospitaller complex and not within the Frankish hospital (which was used for other purposes).[34] It seems that Saladin's hospital was located either in the Church of S. Maria Major[35] or in the Church of S. Maria Latina. On the grounds of one of these, a women's hospital apparently once resided, which functioned in a format similar to that of the central hospital of the Knights of St. John. Thus the establishment of a Muslim hospital did not require a special infrastructure.

In summary, it can be stated with certainty that Saladin's hospital was located in the area where the Hospital of the Knights of St. John operated during the Crusader Period. However, it was accommodated in only a part of the Hospitaller complex, and its activity was more limited as compared to that of the institution that operated during the Frankish Period. From the information available it emerges that Saladin and his successors utilized the Hospitaller property for additional purposes besides the hospital; one part served as the residence of the rulers of the city, another section became a prison and the Mosque of 'Umar, while an additional hall served as a hostel for Muslim mystics (Zawiyat al-Dargah).[36] Likewise it appears that the climax of activity at the al-Bimaristan al-Salahi was reached only during the time of Saladin and the beginning of the Ayyubid dynasty.

The Knights of St. John's Hospital continued to function for a short time after Saladin's conquest of Jerusalem. According to one account, ten Hospitaller brothers remained on the site for about a year, tending the Frankish sick who were left behind.[37]

With the surrender of Jerusalem to Frederich II as part of the Tel 'Ajul-Jaffa treaty, the Hospitaller building complex returned to the Franks for fifteen years. This same building also accommodated the Kaiser when he

---

[32] Mujir al-Din, II, p. 53.
[33] Mujir al-Din, II, p. 47.
[34] Richard, Jerusalem, p. 71.
[35] Richard, Jerusalem, p. 77.
[36] Frenkel, Establishment, p.32; Burgoyne, p. 598.
[37]Richard, Jerusalem, p. 77.

visited Jerusalem.[38] Even before that, some of the Muslim and Jewish residents had abandoned the fortified city.[39] There is no information about what happened to the al-Bimaristan al-Salahi during that period and whether it continued to function as a hospital after the city was restored to Muslim hands in 1244. Although the hospital Waqf is mentioned many times during the Mamluk period, we have no conclusive account of the activity of the al-Bimaristan al-Salahi as a distinctly medical institution. In contrast there are many accounts from that period about the re-populating of the hospital complex of the Hospitallers and transforming it into a center of accommodations for Christian pilgrims in Jerusalem.[40]

Physicians in Jerusalem during the Ayyubid period

Saladin's deliberate cultivation of Jerusalem as a city sacred to Islam on the one hand, and his personal relationship with the medical sciences on the other were the two major factors that attracted many physicians to the city. In the list of physicians drawn up (Section II, items no. 11-21), there are some ten physicians who were active during the Ayyubid Period in Jerusalem.[41] Some of them took advantage of the possibility of visiting the city and stopping at its holy sites. Other physicians made use of the favorable conditions that had been created, thanks to Saladin's policy of developing the city and making it an important center. The arrival of physicians in Jerusalem is also connected to the demand for trained doctors, associated with the development of a system of court physicians. This policy attracted physicians of many religions: Muslims and Jews along with Eastern Christian doctors who practiced medicine in Jerusalem from earlier times. It is especially surprising to note that among those coming to Jerusalem were also renowned physicians and herbalists, some of them preeminent in their field at that time. The origins of these physicians were from various places under Islamic control. Eliyahu ben Zekhariya came from Alexandria, 'Abd al-Latif al-Baghdadai came from Baghdad, Ibn al-Suri came from the city of Tyre, and Abu al-'Abbas al-Nabati and his student Ibn al-Baytar came from Spain. The transformation of Jerusalem into a meeting place for physicians from different regions also helped transmit the different medical traditions that were accepted among the doctors from Spain and North Africa, while during the First Muslim Period the source of the local medical tradition was largely inspired and influenced by Byzantine medical techniques. A considerable number of the physicians who came to Jerusalem served some of the Ayyubid rulers, receiving a regular salary and preferred social standing, and some even passed on their profession and status as an inheritance. Some of the physicians served several different rulers and even wrote books for them. As a result, we have an opportunity to study the status of medicine in al-Sham, and in particular the materia medica that were used there. Information reported by Ibn al-Suri, Abu al-'Abbas al-Nabati, and Ibn al-Baytar teaches much about the use

[38] Prawer, Kingdom, II, p. 93, fn. 51.
[39] Prawer, Colonial, p. 306; Goitein, Jewry, p. 335.
[40] Schein, pp. 145-152.
[41] For the purpose of comparison, Anna-Maria Edde in her study of medicine in the Ayyubid Period brings a list of 56 physicians who served throughout Syria at that time, see: Edde, pp. 103-109.

of a variety of medicinal plants that were found in the Jerusalem region.[42] Furthermore, some of the information about the materia medica used in Jerusalem in earlier periods, as noted by al-Tamimi, was preserved only by virtue of its being emulated by physicians of the Ayyubid Period.[43] At least in this field of medicine, the written literature on herbal medicine, we can state that during this period it reached its peak in terms of quality and popularity as this was reflected in the original treatises written by the prominent medical personalities previously mentioned.

In the chart below appear the names of some of the physicians who were active in Jerusalem during a specific period, even though their major activity was in the service of the sultans outside of the city. In the case of Ibn al-Baytar, a physician who used to full advantage the opportunities that presented themselves in the service of the country in order to enrich his own knowledge, there is no clear-cut evidence that he practiced medicine in Jerusalem, but his personal descriptions of the medicines from this region leave no doubt that he did visit the city.

Physicians in Jerusalem who served the Ayyubid sultanate

Name of physician	Name of sultan
Eliyahu ben Zekhariya	al-Kamil ?
Abu Zekri ben Eliyahu	al-'Aziz 'Utman, al-Mu'azzam 'Isa
Muwaffaq al-Din Ya'qub ibn Siqlab	al-Mu'azzam 'Isa
Rashid al-Din Abu Sa'ed Ibn Yaqub ibn Siqlab	al-Mu'azzam 'Isa, al-Kamil, al-Nasir Daud
Sadid al-Din Abu Mansur Ibn Ya'qub ibn Siqlab	al-Nasir Daud
Rashid al-Din ibn al-Suri	al-'Adil, al-Mu'azzam 'Isa, al-Nasir Daud
Ibn al-Baytar	al-Kamil, al-Nasir Daud
Nagm al-Din ibn al-Labudi	al-Mansur Ibrahim, al-Salih Najm al-Din Ayyub

[42] Amar, Ibn al-Baytar, pp. 49-76; Amar, Herbalist, pp. 235-239.
[43] Amar, Ibn al-Baytar, . 51; Amar, Tradition, pp. 24-25.

The Jewish physicians

According to the account of Yehuda Al-harizi who visited Jerusalem in 1218, Saladin encouraged the Jews to immigrate to Jerusalem.[44] Close to the Muslim conquest of the city (1187) there was a heterogeneous Jewish population in the city which had come from different areas to the east: Ashkelon, Egypt, and Yemen, and from farther points of dispersal in North Africa and western Europe.[45] Some of those who came to settle in Jerusalem were physicians who also enjoyed a high standing in the Jewish community. These physicians were engaged in the practice of medicine in Jerusalem, and some of them joined the system of court physicians of the Ayyubid sultans. One example par excellence of this phenomenon is Eliyahu ben Zekhariya (also known as Abu al-Faraj), the judge, whose family came from Egypt. He lived with his wife and three sons in Jerusalem for a long period around the time of Saladin's conquest of the city. He apparently served as an eye doctor to Malik al-Kamil.[46] Although he is not referred to by his field of specialization, there is mention of his son being an eye-doctor and of his son's request that the father prepare eye medications. His two sons were also involved in the practice of medicine. Abu zekri was an eye doctor and worked in Egypt and Jerusalem as a physician to the rulers al-'Aziz and Malik al-Mu'azzam. Another son was a physician or a physician's assistant who died in the city of Acre and was brought to Haifa for burial.[47]

The Eastern Christian physicians

Following Saladin's conquest of Jerusalem, the Latinate religious hegemony disappeared and the local Eastern Christian community of long-standing again found itself under Muslim rule.[48] As in the pre-Crusader era, it is hard to separate Muslim medicine from Eastern Christian medicine. In Jerusalem the Eastern Christian population had a deeply-rooted local medical tradition that had begun back in the Byzantine Period. The Ayyubid policy regarding the status of medicine encouraged the Eastern Christians to take an active role in the medical system in Jerusalem, as a continuation of their traditional role during the First Muslim and Crusader periods. This was reflected first and foremost in the Christian physicians serving the Ayyubid rulers. The clearest example of this, containing all the hallmarks of the phenomenon of court physician, is Muwaffaq al-Din Ya'qub ibn Siqlab. After Saladin captured Karak (ca. 1188), Yaq'ub ibn Siqlab, still a young man, turned to Damascus to the physician Muwaffaq al-Din As'ad Ibn al-Mutran, a Christian doctor who had converted to Islam and served as his mentor and adviser. When he saw him dressed in blue clothes, in the style of the Frankish physicians, Ibn al-Mutran advised Ya'qub to change his attire as a condition for fitting into the medical profession among Muslims in the country. He did not stop with this

[44] Ya'ari, Travels, p. 67.
[45] Prawer, Colonial, pp. 293-312.
[46] Goitein, Jewry, pp. 322-323, fn. 8.
[47] Goitein, Jewry, pp. 260-275, 327-332; Motzkin, p. 344.
[48] Rose, pp. 189-192.

recommendation but actually sent him silken garments, which was the accepted attire among the local physicians.[49]

The story about Ya'qub ibn Siqlab's attire when he arrived in Damascus attests to the fact that the Eastern doctors in Jerusalem had adopted the customs of the Franks, and with the change in rule, they succeeded in quickly becoming part of the new order, which received them with open arms. For some of the Christian physicians, becoming involved in the new reality did not stop with merely external changes such as apparel; there were also those who changed their religion and demonstrated unqualified loyalty to Islam. That was the case with Ibn al-Mutran. Saladin appreciated this greatly, and made him a confidant, promoting him almost to the rank of vizier.[50]

Ya'qub ibn Siqlab, the protege of Ibn al-Mutran, was a Christian born in Jerusalem, who served as physician to the Ayyubid sultan al-Malik al-Mu'azzam 'Isa (ruled 1218-1228). He practiced medicine in Jerusalem together with another Christian physician named Abu Mansur.[51] He handed both his profession and his position down to his sons. One son, Rashid al-Din Abu Sa'ed served different Ayyubid rulers: al-Mu'azzam (ruled 1218-1228) and from 1234, was physician to al-Kamil, finally serving for nine years as physician to al-Salih Najm al-Din Ayyub (1240-1249). In the end he even wrote one of his medical treatises. [52] The other son of Ya'qub ibn Siqlab was Sadid al-Din Abu Mansur who served in Karak as physician to the Ayyubid ruler al-Nasir Daud.[53]

The biography of Muwaffaq al-Din Ya'qub ibn Siqlab teaches us about the nature of medical studies in Jerusalem. During that time, the classical tradition guided the system of medical education and it was the monks serving in monasteries close to Jerusalem who dominated in the teaching of medicine. It was said of Ya'qub ibn Siqlab that he was most proficient in the teachings of Galenus[54] and that he received his medical training at one of the monasteries of the Judean Desert, which taught the various fields of science, among them medicine. One of his teachers was the philosopher-monk of the al-Siq monastery, who came from Antioch. It was told of this monk that he was well-versed in the natural sciences, geometry, arithmetic, and astronomy.[55] The term 'siq' means 'laura' in Latin, and it is reasonable to assume that this monk belonged to the Mar-Saba Monastery, whose populace was renowned and quite important in the region close to Jerusalem. [56] It appears that the Mar-Saba Monastery was involved in the practice of medicine, not just as theory but also giving actual treatment at the hospital located in the monastery. We hear of this monastery

[49] Ibn abi Usaybi'a, p. 654.
[50] Ibn abi Usaybi'a, p. 653.
[51] Ibn abi Usaybi'a, pp. 697-699.
[52] Ibn abi Usaybi'a, pp. 599-600.
[53] Ibn abi Usaybi'a, p. 699.
[54] Ibn abi Usaybi'a, p. 697. (His son, also a physician, completed his training in Galenus' writings in Damascus under the physician Rashid al-Din 'Ali ibn Halifa, the uncle of Ibn abi Usaybi'a, see: op.cit., p. 599.
[55] Ibn abi Usaybi'a, pp. 697-698; Ibn al-Qifti, pp. 378-379.
[56] Kohlberg & Kedar, p. 125.

later in history.[57] More can be learned about the practice of medicine among the Greek Christians from a medical manuscript dating from the thirteenth or fourteenth century which was written in Arabic and located in the library of the Greek Patriarch of Jerusalem.[58]

[57] Raba, p. 90.
[58] Clark, p. 16.

Chapter Six
The Mamluk Period (1260-1517)

The Mamluk conquest of the Land of Israel (1260) represents a turning point in the status of medicine in the Near East and in the lands under Muslim control as a whole. From this time onward most fields of science controlled by Islam began a steady decline, so different from the cultural renaissance and flowering that were taking place in the West. This was a prolonged process which left its imprint on the fourteenth century. From this time onward we find little evidence of prominent Muslim medical practitioners and there is a conspicuous dearth of original medical treatises, in comparison with the Ayyubid Period, and the status of medicine as a science was in a continuous state of regression. A contemporary of that period, Ibn Khaldun, was also of that impression, as he wrote in his book of prefaces to the science of history circa 1377. He wrote "In Islam, too, there have been physicians of surpassing skill, such as for instance, ar-Râzî, al-Majûsî, and Avicenna...In contemporary Muslim cities, the (craft of medicine) seems to have deteriorated because the civilization (population) has decreased and shrunk..."[1]

The process of cultural decline that characterized the Islamic world during the late Middle Ages was exacerbated by another factor that hurt the status of medicine in the Land of Israel, namely, the policy of the Mamluk rule. The Land of Israel was an area of secondary importance to the kingdom whose center was in Egypt. The Mamluk rulers showed little interest or concern for what was happening in the Land of Israel. The apathy of the Mamluk ruler was expressed among other ways in the paucity of initiatives for building and development (except for religious buildings) and indifference to the needs of the populace. This government conducted a policy characterized by passive, uninspired management, along with exploiting the country's resources as a source of revenue for the state coffers. Jerusalem was at a nadir during the Mamluk Period. Its position as a provincial town remote from the centers of political life and the borders of the kingdom were reflected in the fact that no mail route was sent to it, not even indirectly. Its political and administrative status was of the lowest, and it was considered a place of exile for military officers and minor officials who had offended.[2]

One of the leading hallmarks of the Mamluk Period of rule is the building of many religious buildings in Jerusalem, the strengthening of the Waqk's power, and the involvement of clerics in the life of the city. This may be explained by that fact that the Mamluks who were not Muslim in origin wished to demonstrate their piety and fidelity to Islam, and through the consecrated works they created, wished to create monuments to themselves.[3] On the other hand, they did little to improve the urban infrastructure. It is true that during this period several water works were built by the Mamluk rulers, among them public watering troughs and bath-houses; likewise, the aqueduct to Jerusalem was renovated, bringing with it improved living and sanitation

---

[1] Ibn Khaldun, III, pp. 149-150.
[2] Ashtor, pp. 71-116; Friedman, Eretz, pp. 13-15; Drory, Jerusalem, pp. 152-156.
[3] Drory, Impact, pp. 3-4.

conditions for the city's residents.[4] However, the rulers' initiatives were usually sporadic and were the exception rather than a consistent policy, to the extent that the residents of the city were surprised when Sultan Qaitbay (ca. 1480) repaired the aqueduct that supplied water to Jerusalem.[5]

During the Ayyubid and Mamluk periods, the medical studies and professional apprenticeship of the doctors was carried out in mosques or special madrassas.[6] Unlike in the Ayyubid Period, where we are witness to an convening in Jerusalem of scholars and holding studies in the various disciplines of science[7], during the Mamluk Period there is no information about the study of medicine in Jerusalem, and most of the references are to Egypt. Even the three medical schools established in Damascus in the Middle Ages were also closed down at the end of the Mamluk period.[8]

At the beginning of the Mamluk Period, as during the Ayyubid period, the office of "head of the physicians" ("Ra'is al-atibba") included Egypt, the Land of Israel, and Syria (al-Sham). An example of this is Ibrahim Ibn Abu al-wash Ibn Rashid (d. 1309), a Christian who achieved the status of patriarch, and because of his appointment as head of the physicians and personal physician to Sultan Baibars was forced to convert to Islam.[9] Later, with the reshaping of the Mamluk regime, Greater Syria alone had three people who bore the title "head of the physicians" "head oculist"(Ra'is al-kahhalin), and "head surgeon" (Ra'is al-garaihiyyin). However, their status was limited and they were subordinate to the viceroy (na'ib) in Damascus.[10]

In Jerusalem itself there is no mention of the position of "head of the physicians", because the city held an inferior administrative standing as compared with the viceroys in Gaza and Safad. In contrast, a Waqf document form 1393 mentions Qadi Sharaf al-Din Abu al-Ruh 'Isa as the one responsible for Saladin's Hospital (Bimaristan al-Salahi)[11], except that this appointment was of a religious-administrative nature rather than a professional appointment, as someone who also served as head of the Hanqaht al-Salahiya and many other Waqf properties.[12] The al-Salahiya Hospital is mentioned in some twenty documents of the Waqf in Jerusalem during the Mamluk Period.[13] Also serving at the hospital were a surgeon and an eye doctor.[14] One document from 1394 tells of a woman named Zainab bint yusuf ibn Badr, whose personal effects were

[4] Klein-Franke, pp. 129-130; Drory, Emir, pp. 195-204; Salama & Zilberman, pp. 92-93 .
[5] Drory, Jerusalem, pp. 170-171.
[6] Behrens-Abousif, p. 8.
[7] Ibn abi Usaybi'a, pp. 688-689, 694 on the physician al-Baghdadi.
[8] Shtrauss, II, p. 173.
[9] 'Asqalani, I, p. 77.
[10] Al-Qalqsandi, IV, p. 194. At times the position of "Head of the physicians" was divided between two physicians, see: Sakhawi, IV, p. 36.
[11] Little, Catalogue, p. 10.
[12] On Sharaf al-Din, see: Little, Documents, pp. 199-200. He died in 1395, after an attack of abdominal spasms, see: Ibn Qadi, I, p. 565.
[13] See: Little, Importance, p. 219. About a person who dedicated his property after death, see op. Cit., p. 212; Little, Catalogue, no. 204, p. 203, documents form 1377 that deals with the dedication of fruits of the orchard to the waqf of al-Bimaristan al-Salahi; Burgoyne, p. 66.
[14] Lutfi, p. 307; Burgoyne, p. 62. Neither mentions the exact source of information or additional details.

inventoried when she was admitted to the hospital. The document deals with a legal discussion of the money and other possessions that she claimed she had deposited with the hospital's eye doctor, who denied the story. For our purposes, what is important is the fact that the hospital provided medical and nursing care also to women, almost certainly in a ward separate from the men. It likewise provides information about an orderly patient admission procedure that included a detailed inventory of personal effects.[15] This is similar to the admission procedure at the St. John's Hospital of the Hospitaller Order in Jerusalem which operated in the same region, as reflected in the account provided by an anonymous source from approximately 1180.[16]

However, besides the Waqf documents, there is no other source of information describing the activity of the hospital in Jerusalem. This is in marked contrast to documentation pointing out other hospitals in the Land of Israel: in Safad, Gaza, and Hebron[17]. The absence of any mention of a hospital in Jerusalem in the Mamluk historiographic literature may be interpreted as an indication that the institution that is not worthy of mention, medically speaking. In other words, the al-Bimaristan al-Salahi and the activities of its Waqf continued as a religious institution of philanthropy that provided medical services, apparently of low quality. In any case, this institution must have ceased operations temporarily, as a result of the damage caused by the earthquake of 1458.[18] Possible support for this theory may be found in the treatise written by Mujir al-Din who notes that the minaret of Zawiyat al-Dargah (attached to the hospital) was partially destroyed in the earthquake that occurred that year.[19] The same source also mentions a Muslim sheikh named Muhmad ibn 'Abed a-Rahaman who died in 1487 "in the hospital of Jerusalem".[20]

As to the materia medica sold in Jerusalem, there are several isolated pieces of information such as the receipt for a drug sold in Jerusalem[21] or a list of spices and medicines sold in Mamluk Jerusalem " 'Attar" (the name for a perfume or seller of perfume, spices, or healing materials) in the market called Suq al-Salahiyya.[22], better known as 'Suq al-'Attarin.[23] Among the products mentioned are: licorice root, lotus fruit (sidr), saffron, sumac, and alum. One merchant named al-Hajj Abu Bakr sold spices such as musk, rosemary, cloves, and coconut. Most of the healing drugs referred to are local, but the last two mentioned (coconut and clove) came from southeast Asia and tell of a lively trade in medicinal drugs. One of the documents mentions a Muslim " 'Attar" and notes that the bottles in his shop belonged to a Jew, which shows that there was a

[15] See document no. 615, brought in full in Richard, Jerusalem, pp. 80-82.
[16] Adington, Hospital, pp. xi-xii.
[17] The hospital in Safad: 'Asqalani, I, p. 522; Ibn Katir, XIV, p. 187. In Gaza: al-'Umari, p. 142. In Hebron: Yadin, p. 103.
[18] 'Isa, Tarikh, p. 231.
[19] Mujir al-Din, II, p. 49. See the discussion of the date of repair of the minaret of the Mosque of 'Umar which was apparently destroyed in this earthquake, see: Burgoyne, p. 568.
[20] Mujir al-Din, II, p. 253. Also in a document from 1392 there is mention of a man who died in the hospital, see: Richard, Jerusalem, p. 79.
[21] Little, Importance, p. 214.
[22] See: on the shop of Yusuf Ibn Ibrahim Abi Hassan al-'Attar al-Misri, in: Little, Catalogue, p. 211; Frenkel, Endowing, p. 78 fn. 62. The waqf documents mention several other personalities who bore the nickname " 'Attar" in the middle of the fourteenth century, see: Ahmad al-'Attar, Little, Catalogue, pp. 40, 294. The two brothers, Ahmad and 'Ali, sons of Yusuf al-'Attarain, op.cit., p. 285.
[23] Lutfi, pp. 292-293.

partnership between them.[24] The spice market in Jerusalem where the Jews sold their wares is mentioned in the early Ottoman period.[25]

The lowly status of medicine in Jerusalem during the Mamluk period is established in several sources. We may begin with the problematic source, that scholars have been guarded about using. One of the tales of the "Thousand and One Nights"tells of a prince Zau al-Makan who while visiting his sister in Jerusalem fell mortally ill. The residents of Jerusalem collected money to send him to the hospital in Damascus. In the end he was treated by the engineer at the bathhouse who used various drugs and foods, rosewater, violet, and lotus fruit, sugar, and chickens.[26] While this tale contains a certain measure of legend and is difficult to date, it yet contains realistic elements that may reflect the reality of the late Middle Ages (apparently the fourteenth century), as we see in other stories in this rich collection. We are familiar with the use of these drugs in Jerusalem in other periods as well. What is most interesting is that the patient was sent to the hospital in Damascus rather than to the one in Jerusalem. If the information is reliable, then here is proof that the functioning of the hospital in Jerusalem and the level of medical services at that time were poor, to the extent that the seriously ill were compelled to travel distances to the hospital in Damascus. The distancing of Jerusalem from the center of administrative activity also brought about the immigration of trained physicians to Egypt. An example of this is 'Isma'il ibn Ibrahim al-Muqaddasi (i.e., the Jerusalemite) who had an extensive knowledge of medicine and was considered a skilled physician. He moved to Egypt and lived there for an extended period until he was nicknamed "al-Misri" i.e. the Egyptian.[27] Jerusalem was left with no prominent physicians. We learn from other sources that the few physicians and pharmacists who lived in Jerusalem were not professional, as evidenced by R. Elija of Massa in his letter from Jerusalem of circa 1438:

> "So that you may know: people here earn their living by carpentry...and perfumery and are not trained in the craft of pharmacy and syrups and other things worthy of craft, rather just sit and sell. It is superfluous to say that in the craft of medicine, they are all donkeys..."[28]

Except for these crumbs of information there are no sources to provide information on medicine in the land of Israel. One might say that the vast body of Mamluk historiographic literature written from an Egyptian viewpoint ignored almost completely what was happening in the land of Israel. It would seem that the silence of the Egyptian sources regarding the position of the physician in our region is additional proof of the inferior standing of medicine in the land of Israel, particularly in Jerusalem during the Mamluk Empire.

---

[24] Little, Documents, p. 193.
[25] Moses Basola in Ya'ari, Travels, p. 148. Also in the description of Safad he notes that the Jews had many shops where they sold spices brought to the city from Damascus, op. cit. p. 138.
[26] Rivlin, pp. 551-556.
[27] 'Asqalani, I, p. 387.
[28] Hacker, Elija, p. 259; Ya'ari, Igrot, p. 88.

The sources are likewise silent regarding the status of the medical profession in the local Eastern church, and we can guess that in the Mamluk Period it was in a continuous state of decline. This assumption is based on the fact that from the Mamluk Period onward there are no sources available that refer to the medical services provided by the monks. Furthermore, one cannot ignore the historical reality whereby the Eastern Christian community in Jerusalem was experiencing a process of internal disintegration; a number of communities disappeared while others shrank. Most of the residents of Jerusalem and environs were Muslims, and the number of Christians was small.[29] This is in addition to the process of Islamization that characterized the Land of Israel in general during the Mamluk Period, causing a weakening of the Christian influence.[30] The termination of medical services in the monasteries is attested to by the account of the Russian traveler Agrefenii (ca. 1370). On his visit to the Monastery of Mar-Saba, he noted that near the church there was a large hospital building but that in his time, it was already deserted.[31]

The Fransiscans on Mt. Zion had a hospital for pilgrims headed by Baptista of Lubeck, a physician of German extraction who was sent to serve in Jerusalem at the end of the fifteenth century.[32] This is in addition to the many nursing and philanthropic institutions operated by the various Latin organizations in the late Middle Ages. In effect, beginning in the fourteenth century, the Fransiscans began to undertake all of the functions previously filled in Jerusalem by the military orders in caring for the pilgrims. A hostel was built in the fourteenth century on the foundations of the Crusader al-Maristan complex which served until the second half of the fifteenth century as the central and exclusive accommodation for pilgrims.

The hostel was actually situated on part of the Hospitaller hospital complex.[33] At the time of Ludolf von Suchem (ca. 1340) the hostel could accommodate approximately one thousand people, similar to its days of glory during the Crusader Period. The pilgrims were required to pay for all the accommodations they received.[34] However, during the days of Felix Fabri (1483) the building was half destroyed and could only accommodate some four hundred pilgrims.[35] These sources and the descriptions of other pilgrims do not mention any medical treatment and it would seem that the hostel only provided lodging accommodations.

The sources mention eight physicians (see Section II, items 23-30) who were active in Jerusalem throughout the Mamluk Period. In addition Pietro Casola in 1494 mentions a Jewish physician[36] who was trained in Italy. Another physician, R. Shem-Tov Ibn Fulaya Haspharadi wished to go to the Land of Israel in 1416

---

[29] Rose, pp. 190-192.
[30] Amar, Islam, pp. 251-258.
[31] Raba, p. 90.
[32] Arce, p. 123; Felix Fabri, PPTS, 9-10, p. 113.
[33] Schein, pp. 142-156. On Antonio de la Cour who was "guardianus Hospitalis Jherusalem" (in charge of the hospitals in Jerusalem) see op. cit., p. 151.
[34] PPTS, 12, pp. 106-107.
[35] PPTS, 7-8, p. 395. The building was apparently destroyed by the earthquake in 1458.
[36] Casola, p. 271.

when he was 63 years old, and it is not clear if he succeeded in realizing his wish.[37] As for people who practiced medicine in Jerusalem, one may also learn of their profession from their nicknames, for example: a person named Jaraihi ('surgeon') and two personages named Kahhal ('eye doctor') are mentioned in the years 1393-1394; one of them is a Muslim named Muhmad al-Misri and the other, a Christian named 'Ali IbnYusuf.[38] In summary the information on physicians in Jerusalem during the Mamluk Period – otherwise so rich in sources – is relatively scant, although it is certain that additional physicians worked there. Documentation in that area is lacking.

[37] Hacker, Connections, pp. 114, 133-137.
[38] Lutfi, p. 307; Burgoyne, p. 62; Little, Catalogue, pp. 165, 266.

Chapter Seven
Medicine in Jerusalem during the Ottoman Period
(until the end of the 18th century)

At the beginning of the Ottoman Period, the community in the Land of Israel began to show signs of recovery. For nearly half a century the country demonstrated appreciable demographic and economic growth, the product of the vigorous rule of a new, efficient administration. Thus, for example, during the reign of Sultan Suleiman the Magnificent (1520-1566) Jerusalem achieved a momentum of building and expansion of construction for both secular and sacred purposes. Among the public works instituted in Jerusalem for the welfare of its residents were an improvement in the water supply to the city, new watering troughs, and renovations in the "Sultan's Pool".[1] This also had a concomitant impact, at least for a certain time, in improving the level of sanitation and health in Jerusalem. The new conditions that were created in the beginning of the Ottoman Period also brought growth to the Jewish community in the land, primarily the result of waves of immigration from all over the Jewish world. Especially noteworthy is the immigration from Spain and Portugal which had a strong influence on the ethnic and cultural character of the Jewish community in the land of Israel.

One distinctive feature of this study is the prominent presentation of the subject of Jewish physicians in Jerusalem. This is primarily due to the multiplicity of research in Israel which focuses on the history of the Jewish people and their settlement there during the Ottoman Period and less on the Muslim and Christian communities. However, it would not be remiss in the context of this study to adopt the general proposition that the state of the Jewish community in Jerusalem at the beginning of the Ottoman Period represents a faithful reflection of the overall social and demographic reality. In other words, a considerable part of the information we have on the condition of medicine and the status of physicians in Jerusalem as it relates to the Jews in many studies represents a reliable reflection also of the Muslim and Christian physicians and a description of the status of medicine in general in Jerusalem.

The physicians

Knowledge about the physicians in Jerusalem at the end of the Mamluk period and the beginning of the Ottoman period until the end of the eighteenth century is gleaned from sporadic scraps of information that appear in the various written sources. A large portion of the information is drawn from documents of the Muslim court in Jerusalem.

[1] Heyd, Documents, pp. 146-150; Cohen, Jewish, p. 220; Salama & Zilberman pp. 91-106; Singer pp. 190-197.

From these sources we know of over fifty personages from Jerusalem by their full names who bore the title "physician". However, these physicians can not be seen as one group with uniform characteristics. Some of them were natives of Jerusalem while some came in order to be buried there at the end of their life. Others of these physicians came on pilgrimages from various places in the world and worked in the city for several years. In the seventeenth century many Christian physicians visited Jerusalem as pilgrims, among them Gabriel Bremond of Marseilles (1660), Angelo Legrenzi of Venice (1673-1674), and the Italian physician Francis Gemelli Careri (1693).[2] One must also mention the physicians, nursing brothers, and pharmacists who were sent to serve in Jerusalem by the Franciscans.[3]

In addition to the names of known physicians, the sources also refer to physicians from Jerusalem without mentioning them by name. Thus, for example, the Italian traveler Cornelio Magni who visited Jerusalem in 1677, tells of a Portuguese Jew who served in his day as a physician in Jerusalem and whom the Turkish authorities consulted professionally.[4] The Franciscan monk Elzear Horn attests that he himself used the services of an elderly Ashkenazic Jewish physician who was a graduate of the University of Padua in Italy and who resided at that time in Jerusalem. That was on 8.8. 1729 and according to Horn, this physician died a short time afterwards, which cast a heavy pall on the Jewish community, and he was buried in the Valley of Jehosophat on 24.12. 1729.[5] All the signs point to identifying this physician as Tobias Cohen.

Furthermore, we have information about physicians who lived in Jerusalem for only a short period in order to visit relatives or for business purposes, such as Raphael Morino "the eminent physician philanthropist" of Alexandria who forwarded money for the Jews of Jerusalem in 1652.[6] There are physicians who were preparing to immigrate to the land of Israel and particularly Jerusalem, and there are clear accounts of these who were not able to realize their goal. As an example, we may cite the case of R. Yoseph Hamitz who was ordained as rabbi by R. Yehuda Aryeh of Modina and by the rabbinical sages of Venice. He attended the University of Padua, where he was awarded the title of "Doctor of Medicine and Philosophy" in 1624 and was called "an expert physician. In 1647 he decided to immigrate to Jerusalem and to establish a yeshiva [Talmudic academy] where sages from Italy would study but due to various circumstances, he was unable to realize his plan.[7] Another figure was Dr. Gordon Yoseph of Lita who was qualified in medicine at the University of Padua in 1732 and also engaged extensively in the study of the *kabbalah*. Some twenty years later he began concrete preparations to immigrate to the Land of Israel to study Torah there but this never

2 Schur, Community p. 397, 399, 403.
3 Arce pp. 117-120, 325; table no. 2.
4 Schur, Community p. 400.
5 Horn pp. 179-180.
6 Benayahu, Generation, p. 179, 314.
7 Benayahu, Generation, pp. 298-300, fn. 15.

came to fruition.[8] These personalities, although they never immigrated to the land of Israel, are typical of a cross-section of physicians who were active in Jerusalem.

The medical staff at the St. Saviour Franciscan Monastery in Jerusalem

There is no complete and systematic documentation available about the medical staff that served at the Franciscan Order in the land of Israel in general and in Jerusalem in particular. The information brought here is fragmentary and in the main relates to figures who died in Jerusalem. In other words, only those who were documented in the Jerusalem Franciscan death certificates are referred to here and it is certain that in the17th-18th century a larger medical staff was employed there. In effect, apart from this data, we have hardly any other information about the medical staff's mode of work. The list consists of seven physicians, eight nursing brothers, and nine staff members trained in a profession akin to pharmacy (some of these individuals worked as both physicians and pharmacists).

Table no. 2: The medical staff at the Franciscan Monastery in Jerusalem

Name (transliterated from the original record)	Year of visit/activity	Function
Pacificus de Pariana	1651	Pharmacist
Joseph de Ottaviano	1652-1676	Physician
Franciscus de Genua	1654-1660	Nursing brother
Cherubinus de Sancta Lucia	1658	Nursing brother
Joseph de Reate	1658	Pharmacist
Iohannes Antonius de Antico	1672-1674	Nursing brother
Iohannes Angelus de Saravalle	1681	Pharmacist
Matthaeus de Valle Agni	1681	Pharmacist
Honorius de Alessano	1683-1687	Pharmacist
Antonius Menzani de Cuna	1686-1729	Physician & pharmacist
Petrus de Zalana	1687-1736	Nursing brother
Nicolaus de Luca	1697-1713	Nursing brother
Angelus de Prisciano	1704-1730	Physician & pharmacist
Iohannes Gallego	1705-1744	Physician
Sanctus de Venetiis	1711- 1713	Physician
Venantius de Orbassano	1751- 1754	Nursing brother
Hieronymous de Marostica	1752-1753	Pharmacist's apprentice
Laurentius de Manarola	1774-1782	Nursing brother
Franciscus López	1788-1813	Physician & pharmacist
Didacus Marchiori de Nomi	1745-1749	Nursing brother
Antonius Paláu	1784-1790	Physician

* According to Arce, pp. 117-120, 324-325.

[8] Gelber, p. 356.

The status of physicians

Physicians in the Ottoman Period belonged to an elite social class. As befitted their eminent status, they were distinguishable by their unique garb and they may have even been allowed to wear a sword. In the event that this practice was also accepted in our region, this was a privilege conferred only upon those physicians who worked in the public service on behalf of the imperial administration. R. Moses Hajiz, a hakham (rabbi) from the land of Israel in the first part of the eighteenth century discussed the subject of whether Jewish physicians were likewise permitted to act in this manner:

"For it is the practice of every expert physician that he wear the special garb that marks him as a skilled physician and he is permitted to wear it ...for even the Jewish physicians wear it. And in these counties where they used to gird a sword at the waist, Jewish physicians may also do so during the weekdays, but not on the Sabbath in any way."[9]

Most of the Jewish physicians served as leaders of the Jewish community and as its representatives to the authorities, and some were among its preeminent Torah scholars. Some of these personalities actually practiced medicine while others had medical training but did not engage in actual practice.

Despite the paucity of material, one may learn several important facts about the origin of the physicians, their professional training, and more generally, about the nature of medicine in Jerusalem.

Professional training

Several types of "physicians" operated in Jerusalem.[10] The first type was the qualified physician who is known in the sources as "distinguished physician", or "expert physician" who studied at an accredited medical establishment. This category recognizes only physicians of the male gender. Among the "distinguished physicians" there are also doctors who served under other "distinguished physicians" known in their field, and who were certified by dint of their experience and practical studies. A doctor's practical study was carried out at a hospital.[11] There were medical schools only in the centers of large cities in the Ottoman Empire. One such accredited medical establishment, for example, is the imperial school attached to the court of the sultan at Galata Saray in Istanbul which Jews also attended. Physicians who completed their course of study received an official appointment from the government. In the writ of appointment was a definition of the physicians' field of expertise, for example, surgeon, eye doctor, and intuitive

---

[9] Hajiz, Responsa No. 262, p. 129.
[10] For a classification of physicians in late nineteenth century, Jerusalem , see: Droyanov, p. 48.
[11] Murphey, p. 381.

physiognomy.[12] Physicians with all of these fields of specialized training served in Jerusalem, and a physician who had not completed his professional specialization was not permitted to practice, until he had passed an examination and received official certification.

The physicians were affiliated in a professional association (guild) headed by the "Head of the physicians in Jerusalem" who was appointed by the authorities, among other functions, to maintain the professional standards of physicians in his city and to supervise them and ensure the continuing study of physicians who had not yet completed their professional training.[13]

The "distinguished physicians" who came from central and western Europe received their training at different universities, particularly at Padua. We are witness to a significant transformation in the study of medicine at the prominent universities in Europe, a shift to the principles of scientific empiricism, which represented the precursors of modern medicine as we know it today.[14] It should be noted that the University of Padua and later Leyden were considered liberal academic institutions with a tolerant attitude toward students of other religions and nationalities. Due to discriminatory practice, the Jews who studied at the universities of Europe were awarded the title of "Magister" upon completion of their studies. This degree was largely a vocational diploma that qualified its bearer to engage in the practice of medicine, sometimes with certain restrictions. Beginning in the sixteenth century, the way was opened for Jews to earn the title of "Doctor" which also made it possible for them to teach at the universities and to win the privileges and financial benefits that were the reward of the office-holders and functionaries who worked in the public service. Study at the university was attended by obstacles and the requirement to pay particularly large sums of money. One of the limitations was religious; the title of doctor was conferred in a religious ceremony that involved taking the doctor's oath according to a religious Catholic version. Later the Jews were offered the possibility of receiving a "secular" title of doctor that was awarded by representatives of the Emperor. Official documents show that at first, the number of Jews who were awarded the title of doctor at the universities of Europe was relatively small, but the seventeenth century onward, with the lifting of some of the strictures on the Jews, is marked by a steadily increasing number of Jews who are awarded the title.[15]

The second type of physician in Jerusalem was the "folk" practitioner who did not undergo any recognized medical training. These practitioners were usually not mentioned explicitly in the imperial records. This category included women who were engaged in folk medicine. Of special note were the women eye specialists who did not have the formal medical training of the 'eye physicians'; however, many people came to them to utilize their services as healers, whose experience had been proven and brought them their repute.

---

[12] On the types of physicians and of professional specialization in the Ottoman Empire, see: Murphey, p. 382.
[13] Cohen, 16th Century, pp. 268-271; al-'Asali, Wata'iq, pp. 89-91.
[14] Palmer, pp. 100-117, and especially in Smith, Science.
[15] Friedenwald, pp. 221-240; Ruderman, pp. 100-117; Dubnov, pp. 216-219; Kaplan, pp. 65-75; Carpi, pp. 96-130.

The work of the folk practitioners and of the eye specialists in particular was recognized quasi-officially by the authorities, who permitted them to practice their craft, and when they caused damage to any of their patients, they were required to pay compensation, just like the distinguished physicians. One example is the case of an eye specialist by the name of Rena bat Avraham the Jew who was sued in court by a Muslim patient whom she had treated.[16] Other Jewish eye specialists mentioned in the documents of the sixteenth and eighteenth centuries are Lipa bat Ya'akov the Jew[17] and Sara Um Moshe.[18] The eye clinics operated in private houses in the Jewish neighborhood.[19]

The number of physicians in Jerusalem

It is hard to know the overall number of physicians of the various nationalities in Jerusalem at every period. This is because of the lack of data in the research literature. Furthermore, the number of physicians at every period is apparently not related to the size of Jerusalem's population or to the distribution among the different religions. That is because the service of the physicians in Jerusalem as part of the imperial apparatus was determined (besides by decision of the Head of the physicians) by professional rather than ethnic criteria. The number of physicians who worked within the framework of the Franciscan monastery was not uniform and was contingent upon the professional manpower that had been sent to Jerusalem. Thus, in the first third of the eighteenth century, there were four physicians in service[20], nonetheless, there were also periods of time when there was no physician at all at the monastery. In such a situation, the medicines at the Franciscan pharmacy were supplied without a doctor's prescription or by a prescription written by a physician belonging to another ethnic community, including Jews.[21]

In contrast, it is possible to form a general estimate of the number of Jewish physicians. In documents of the Muslim court in Jerusalem there were records of at least twenty Jewish physicians in Jerusalem over the entire course of the sixteenth century [between 1531-1587].[22] If we assume that this is a representative rather than an atypical number, then on the average there were three-four physicians practicing in Jerusalem in every generation. In the Ottoman tax records of 1690 there is mention of three physicians [Hekim] and six pharmacists and drug sellers ['Attarin].[23] R. Gedalya of Siemiatycze notes in 1700 "And the Jews also have several shops in the gentile marketplace such as spice-sellers and the like, but they are few."[24] Seetzen who brings the list of Jewish professionals in Jerusalem in 1806 lists Jewish physicians and ten shops selling

[16] Cohen, 18th Century, p. 328, no. 286, from 1760.
[17] Cohen, 16th Century, p. 310, no. 353, from 1551.
[18] Cohen, 18th Century, p. 326, no. 281, from 1720.
[19] An eye clinic (al-kahhala) in the Jewish neighborhood is mentioned in documents, see: Cohen, 16th Century, p. 286, no. 324, (from 1570); Cohen, 18th Century, p. 382, no. 363, (from 1719); p. 426, no. 412, (from 1715); p. 438, no. 427, (from 1717).
[20] Arce, pp. 118-119.
[21] Horn, pp. 177-179.
[22] Cohen, Jewish, p. 188.
[23] Heyd, Jews, pp. 179-180.
[24] Ya'ari, Travels, pp. 334-335.

spices and medicines.[25] R. Eliezer Bergman also reports that in 1815 Jerusalem had three expert physicians, one of them from Poland and one from Izmir.[26] Further verification of this number can be obtained from a reference to the names of Jewish physicians who were engaged in the practice of medicine in Jerusalem throughout the eighteenth century. The list of names reaches approximately ten, an average of three doctors per generation. All of these sources indicate a fairly constant number; in other words, in the sixteenth through the eighteenth centuries, three Jewish physicians on the average were in service. At the same time we presume that the number of Jewish physicians in Jerusalem during these years was greater. The figures pointing to three physicians on the average is largely based on official data. In other words, the data relates to qualified doctors who were officially recognized by the ruling authorities.

Institutions of healing

The functioning of the institution of the "hospital" in ancient times did not focus exclusively on medical treatment of the sick, as in modern times. The hospital was a welfare institution which functioned, beyond purely medical treatment, as a philanthropic institution engaged in assistance and hospitality, functioning as a soup kitchen, supporting the indigent, abandoned, orphans, and the like. The hospital institution in its broader sense was a familiar one in Jerusalem from earlier periods, and its structure crystallized into this format during the Byzantine period.[27] An extensive description of the hospital institution and the diversified services it provided are mentioned in the Crusader Period. In the Ottoman Period, too, the hospital functioned in the same format, until the arrival of modern medicine to Jerusalem in the nineteenth century.

We read again of the hospital (al-Bimaristan) in Jerusalem beginning in the Ottoman Period and it is not clear if it is still on the same site that there had been a hospital in the Ayyubid and Mamluk periods. In the sixteenth century, one of the documents of the Muslim court refers to a Jewish Karaite physician who worked as a substitute at the hospital.[28] In another document from the end of 1760 there are references to Jews who died at the hospital in Jerusalem whose relatives were exempted from paying burial fees.[29] This was the official hospital for the entire Jerusalem population. The general hospital is a continuation, or more precisely, the renewal of the al-Bimaristan al-Salahi.[30] The hospital complex was dilapidated and every few years, a committee would convene and recommend that it be repaired and renovated. Thus, for example, in documents from 1570 and 1636 there are accounts of an attempt to repair and develop the al-bimaristan which belonged to the waqf of the al-Bimaristan al-Salahi. The documents indicate that the structure was

[25] Seetzen, p. 23.
[26] Bergman, p. 92.
[27] Ashkenazi, Involvement, pp. 43-49.
[28] Cohen, Jewish, p. 189.
[29] Cohen, 18th Century, p. 108, no. 89.
[30] On the waqf of this institution, see: Cohen, Jewish, p. 211; Burgoyne, p. 580.

partially destroyed and included several sub-divisions: a general hospital, a mental hospital, and an eye clinic.[31]

In effect, the medical services in Jerusalem may be classified into three categories: public medicine, community medicine, and private medicine.

Public medicine

The public hospital was supposed to serve the entire population of Jerusalem, without distinction of religion, and it is only natural that it primarily served the Muslim population which represented the majority in the city. This is in addition to the fact that the Jewish and Christian communities had smaller medical institutions of their own. As opposed to the community institutions of medicine that were funded by contributions, the public hospital was supported by the central imperial government or by waqf funds. The physicians who served at this hospital received an appointment and a salary with incentive pay, since Jerusalem was considered a backwater in the Ottoman Empire. Seeing the physician as part of the apparatus designed to serve the general public was reflected in the fact that the physician was not permitted to leave Jerusalem without sufficient reason, and then only with advance permission, and after finding a substitute for his job.[32] A document from 1789 shows that in addition to the various physicians employed by the hospital, someone was also employed to be in charge of the food supply (kalarjia) and another person who was responsible for medicinal potions and drugs (sharabatjia).[33] In a document from 1694 there is reference to the appointment of Sheikh ‘Ali and Sheikh ‘Abed, two learned friars who received money from the al-Bimaristan al-Salahi for reading sura no. 36 every Monday and Thursday.[34] The Muslim faith ascribes many virtues to the reading of this chapter of the Quran which keeps away the angel of death, and it is generally done at a person’s last hour or during the funeral.

Physicians of all ethnic communities were allowed to practice at the public hospital. Some of the physicians were natives of Jerusalem and its environs, while some were sent by the imperial government at Istanbul. This category also included Jews. One example is the Jewish physician Yehia whose writ of appointment (dated 29.10.1564) stated that “he preferred to be a physician in Jerusalem”.[35] It is possible that this physician had relatives in Jerusalem or perhaps he wanted to immigrate there for religious reasons. However, it did not always happen that the Jewish physicians who were sent to work in Jerusalem adjusted successfully to the life of the Jewish community there. In one document of the Muslim court dated 1767 there is mention of a Jewish physician, one Kamil, who was "one of the physicians residing in Jerusalem”. This document

[31] al-‘Asali, Wata’iq, pp. 87-88; Ze’evi, p. 39.
[32] Cohen, 16th Century, p. 268.
[33] al-‘Asali, Wata’iq, pp. 89-90.
[34] al-‘Asali, Wata’iq, p. 90.
[35] Cohen, 16th Century, p. 269, no. 303.

indicates that the relationship between Kamil and his son Amin with the rest of his co-religionists of the Jewish community were less than cordial. The former applied to the central government in Istanbul with a request that it prevent the Jewish community from doing him any injury and their petition was accepted.[36]

Community medicine

In addition to the general, imperial hospital, there were physicians who practiced in private clinics or at the hospital of their own ethnic community.[37] The Jews and Christians preferred, for religious reasons, to use the medical services of their own communities, and the Ottoman government recognized their needs. Besides these, there were apparently Muslim philanthropic institutions which also provided a sort of medical assistance. In the first half of the eighteenth century several European sources mention the Hospital of St. Helena which served as a hospice for the Muslim poor which was maintained by the Ottoman government.[38] [Fig. 16]. This institution is mentioned many times in the nineteenth century and was known as the "Tekiyeh", that is, the soup kitchen.

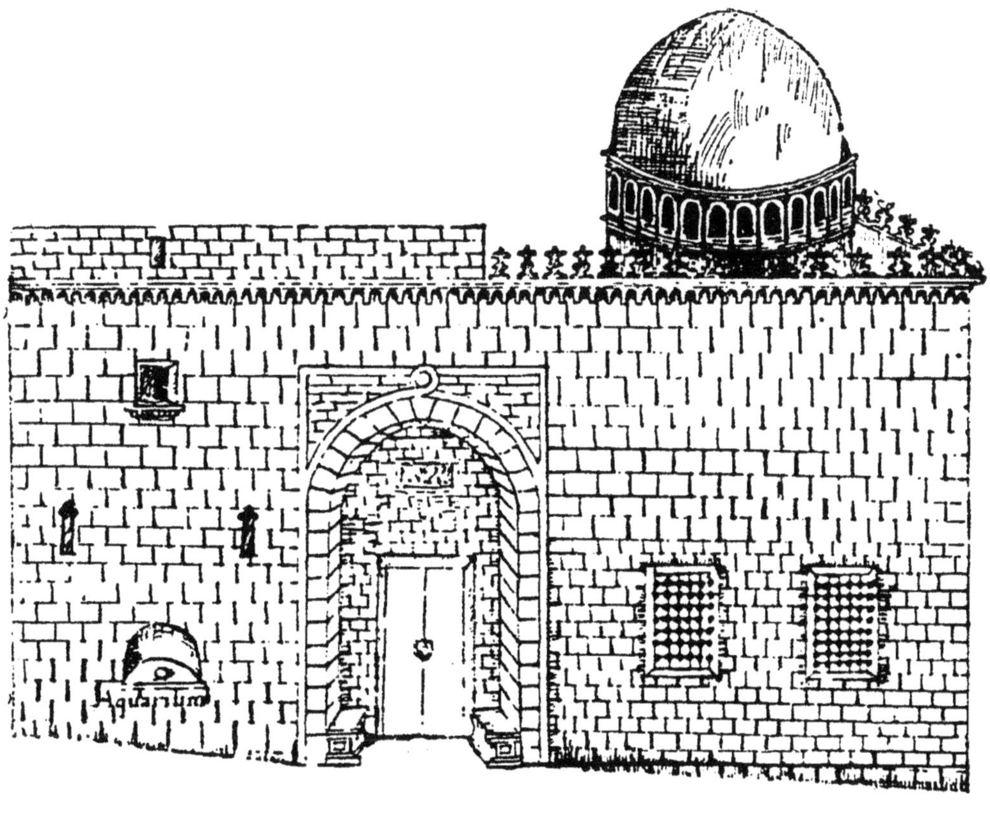

Figure 16: Hospital of St. Helena (according to Horn).

[36] Cohen, 18th Century, pp. 274-275, no. 235.
[37] See: Cohen, Jewish, p. 191.
[38] Horn, pp. 191-193; Hasselquist, p. 135.

In the sixteenth-eighteenth centuries, the Jewish community in Jerusalem had its own house of the sick – bimaristan – where the Jewish sick were treated until they recovered.[39] The Jewish bimaristan was located in the Jewish neighborhood.[40] It seems that the imperial government allowed the building of a separate hospital for the Jews in consequence of its acknowledgement of the halachically-ordained needs and problems that might arise for Jews in a public hospital.

Furthermore, the authorities recognized the Ashkenazic community as a separate entity with its own hospital which served as an almshouse for the sick and needy. In one document from 1579 there is explicit mention of one Avraham ben Natan "who was in charge of the hospital of the Ashkenazic community in the city of Jerusalem".[41] From this source one may deduce that if the Ashkenazic community, which was a minority, had its own hospital, then the Sephardic community must have had a hospital of its own as well. In fact, all of the casual references to the hospital of the Jews in Jerusalem apparently are referring to the hospital of the Sephardic community.

During the Ottoman Period, the Karaite community was considered by the authorities as part of the Jewish community of Jerusalem, even though it had its own separate administrative institutions.[42] It is not clear if they also had their own hospital. Although the Jews did have their own hospital, this does not imply that the Jews did not turn at all to the public hospital. It seems that for difficult and complicated medical procedures such as surgery, the Jews availed themselves of the services of public medicine which were manned by qualified physicians, some of them Jews. At the same time, for milder diseases which did not require specialized skills, they went to the community hospital which was more limited in its budget and the level of professional expertise it could offer.

Bikkur Holim

The Jewish community hospital in Jerusalem was apparently part of the responsibility of the "Kupat Bikkur Holim", (fund for visiting the sick) an institution widely described in Jewish sources of the seventeenth century. In truth this was a social welfare institution which provided welfare and charitable assistance and in particular, support for the indigent sick who were unable to afford private medical care. This institution operated in a similar format in many places throughout the Ottoman Empire as well as in the land of Israel, such as in the city of Safad.[43]

---

[39] Cohen, Jewish, p. 15; Cohen, 18th Century, p. 172, fn. 1, no. 138; p. 176, fn. 3, no. 142.
[40] Cohen, 16th Century, p. 321, no. 366.
[41] Cohen, Jewish, p. 58; Cohen, 16th Century, p. 339, no. 382, regarding the request to renovate the Ashkenazic hospital.
[42] See: Cohen, 18th Century, p. 44.
[43] See: Cooley, on Ex. 21: 18-19, p. 708; Kupfer, pp. 362-363.

R. Refael Mordekhai Malki, who described the state of medicine in Jerusalem, provides a great deal of information relating to the institution of "Bikkur Holim" which was sponsored and supervised by the Jewish community leadership but not funded by it. The institution was supported by charity funds and private donations. The treasurers of the charity funds would collect money every day at a different synagogue. In addition, there were individuals who donated a certain sum weekly, as well as those who were honored in the synagogue with being called up to the Torah and guests who visited the synagogue, in addition to charitable contributions from several Jewish communities in Europe.[44] In example one may cite the case of Hisqiya de Silva, the son-in-law of Refael Malki who was sent to the Spanish-Portuguese community in Amsterdam at the request of the eminent rabbis of Jerusalem to try to raise funds for the community's needs. While carrying out his commission, he gave a speech in Spanish-Jewish (Ladino) in 1691 about the commandment of charity to the sick and other subjects related to the commandment of visiting the sick but he did not connect his speech directly to the institutions of Bikkur Holim in Jerusalem and a request for support by the Jewish community in Amsterdam on behalf of the Jerusalem Jewish residents. [45] With the money collected, the treasurer of the fund would purchase food and medicines and would allocate each sick person a sum based on his needs and the funds available, which was generally quite small.[46]

The main support given by the fund to the sick was in distributing chickens and various syrups (potions made of different flowers and fruit such as roses, sugar, and almonds).[Fig. 17][47] It is interesting that both of these main components are mentioned in a medical document describing the medical service given by the St. John's Hospital in Jerusalem during the Crusader Period.[48]

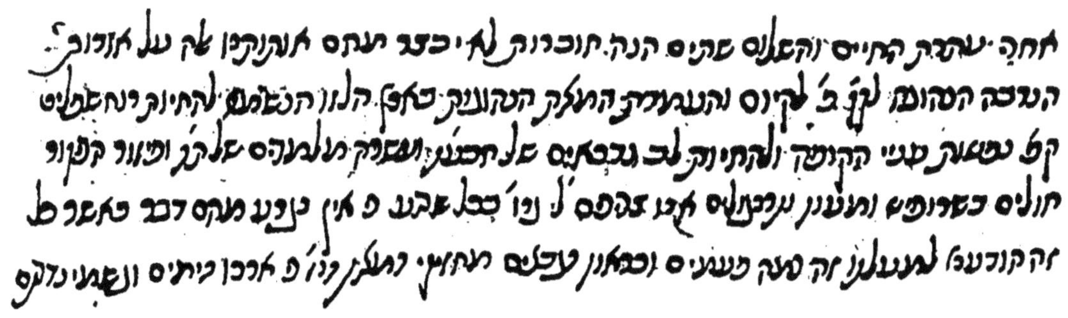

Figure 17: Fragment of a letter written in seventeenth century Jerusalem with a request for assistance for various community needs. Mentioned among others:

"Regarding the donation habitual for the Jewish community here in Jerusalem, in order to uphold and fulfill the commandments of this land to restore the spirit of the down-trodden, 180 souls, dependent on the community funds, and to encourage the indigent Torah scholars, and ten teachers of the young children and to distribute aid to the sick in the form of syrups, and money, and chickens, we require 30 gro. weekly..."

From: A manuscript from the Yellin collection, Jerusalem, National Library, Figure 61 8° letter Figure 108, p. 143.

[44] Malki, pp. 57-58; Rozen, Identity, pp. 152-153.

[45] Tuito, pp. 53-75.

[46] Malki, p. 45; pp. 57-58, 61-62; Rozen, Community, pp. 170-171, 443, letter no. 43.

[47] Malki, p. 58; Yalin, p. 92; Rozen, Community, p. 434, letter no. 36; p. 511, letter no. 108.

[48] Delaville, no. 627. Cf. Goitein, Jewry, p. 324,

The treasurer of the fund was in effect the only medical authority actually engaged in caring for the sick. The absence of a qualified physician in this institution was apparently connected to the lack of funds for paying a physician, since the source of revenue was based on donations rather than the community's coffer. The Bikkur Holim institution was not truly a hospital in the full sense of the word but rather functioned more as a kind of clinic. Incidentally R. Refael Malki who advocated a professional administration of Bikkur Holim contended that an expert physician had never headed it because of the absence of expert physicians in Jerusalem.[49] His words may have reflected the reality of his times, for there is abundant clear-cut evidence that there were qualified physicians in Jerusalem in other generations (see list of physicians appearing in Part II of this book).

There is no information available on an Ashkenazic hospital or sick assistance fund in the seventeenth and eighteenth centuries and it may well be that for lack of proper funding, the Bikkur Holim institution served the entire Jewish population of Jerusalem, Ashkenazic and Sephardic alike.

After the immigration of the students of the Vilna Gaon to Jerusalem in 1809 the influence of the "separatists" in Jerusalem grew, namely those who wished to maintain a community leadership separate from that of the Sephardim and the Hassidim. A consciousness of medical needs was highly developed among this separatist community, and among the students of the Vilna Gaon who immigrated to the land of Israel were individuals with medical knowledge, such as R. Zalman Doktor and R. Hillel Rivlin. As to the establishment of a sick assistance fund in Jerusalem by the separatists, there is confirmed information of this as of 1837, although this institution might have been established even earlier. Eventually this was to become a modern hospital. This institution, too, was funded by contributions, so that existing alongside each other there were two sick assistance societies: separatists and Sephardic-Hassidim which were limited in their abilities to provide proper medical care.[50]

The Franciscan medical institution and the Balm of Jerusalem

We have information from the beginning of the sixteenth century of a special hospital for the Christian community. It seems that most of the Christian population used the services of either the public hospital or of private medicine. Apparently some of the monasteries and Christian institutions around Jerusalem offered their services as well, but we have no information about a Christian institution of healing with a clearly functional apparatus. It is true that in at the end of the Mamluk Period the Franciscans on Mt. Zion had a hospital but it was largely designed to serve pilgrims[51], and it functioned primarily as an institution of

[49] Malki, p. 68.
[50] Freidin, pp. 117-140.
[51] Schein, p. 144; Arce, p. 123, who thinks that the Franciscans began to practice medicine and pharmacology in 1342, when twelve clergymen settled permanently in the land of Israel.

welfare and charity. It would appear that the absence of a proper Christian institution of medicine along with the Christian ideology that one must avoid seeking assistance from Jews and Muslims were factors in the development of the Franciscan institution of healing in Jerusalem during the Ottoman Period.

In the sixteenth century there are references to three healers who arrived in the land of Israel in 1524 for a stay of three years. One was a pharmacist and the other two were nursing brothers.[52] It is not completely clear when the Franciscan institution of St. Saviour was built. The pharmacy is first mentioned in 1620.[53] The monastery possessed a copy of the book of Dioscorides in Mattioli's edition (1501-1577) which was left on the site in 1628 by Cherubino de Mesina for the benefit of the pharmacists' storehouse.[Fig. 18] [54] Indeed, the institution's major role at that time was as a pharmacy rather than a hospital. Even when the hospital was built above the pharmacy, it did not provide service to women and plague victims.[55] The sources cited below and the list of the medical staff that operated at the Franciscan hospital in Jerusalem[56] shows that most of the functionaries had professional training related to nursing and pharmacy rather than clearly medical in nature.

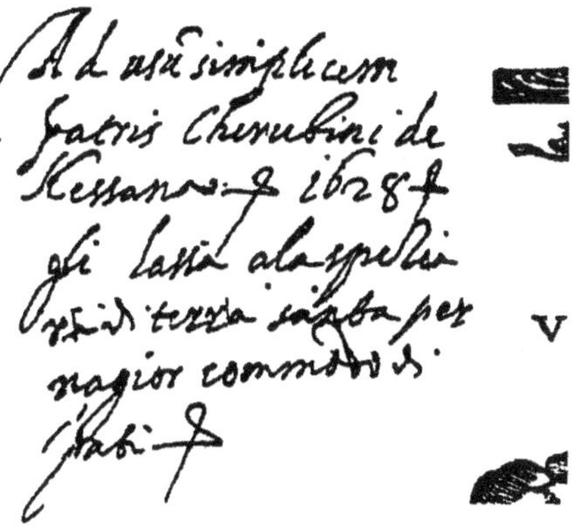

Figure 18: Dedication in a medical book left in 1628 by Cherubino de Mesina for the benefit of the pharmacists' storehouse in Jerusalem.

Elzear Horn, a Franciscan monk of German origin who resided in the Land of Israel between 1724-1744, described at length the pharmacy of the Franciscans, which he claimed was one of the best in the entire Christian world. In the warehouses of this pharmacy one could find a wide variety of drugs: spices, flowers, peels, roots, seeds in glass or wooden jars, oils, perfumes, and precious stones [Fig. 19] The medical materials were purchased with the help of contributions by philanthropists from all over the Christian world, particularly from Venice. The pharmacy included labs with medical and apothecary instruments, such as: distilling equipment and surgical instruments. The pharmacy was administered by two friars, at least one of whom had professional training. The drugs were given with a doctor's prescription, if there was a doctor available. The pharmacists were called upon to demonstrate a high level of proficiency in their work which included recognizing the medical drugs according to characteristics such as hardness, color, weight as well as correctly defining the precise dosage required. The pharmacists had to know how to store the medicines for prolonged periods of time against any possible damage and to seal the jars against evaporation. They had to

[52] Arce, p. 324.
[53] Bagatti, p. 353; Schittny, p. 41.
[54] See in the introduction of Horn, p. 8.
[55] Horn, p. 180.
[56] Arce, pp. 177-120, 325.

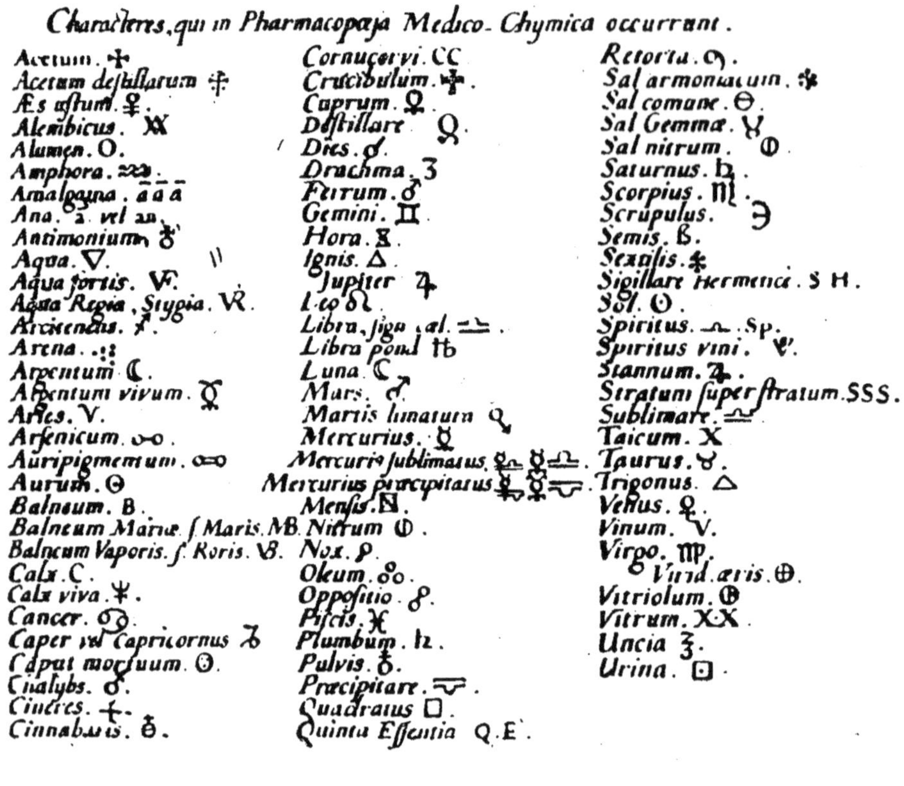

Figure 19: Chart of symbols of materia medica in the Franciscan pharmacy in Jerusalem.

replace them after the expiration time every few months or years, depending on the nature of the medicine. The work of the pharmacist required knowledge of many crafts: distilling, separating, macerating, mixing ingredients, pouring liquids, etc. [57] The medicinal substances were kept in glazed earthenware jars (most, using the maiolica technique) and elaborately adorned with identifying marks of the materia medica. These jars were donated from Italy to the monastery during the period that the pharmacy was in operation and can be dated by a comparative typological analysis and the date stamped on the bottom of some of them. [Fig. 20]. At present one may find at the Monastery of the Flagellation in Jerusalem some 200 pharmacist jars, of the 449 that were catalogued.[58]

Frederich Hasselquist, who visited the land of Israel in 1750, also describes with some emotion the pharmacopoeia of the Franciscans in Jerusalem, which contained a rich storehouse of potions and medicines:

> "It was amazing to see what quantities of the dearest Drugs their magazine contained. All sorts of balsams were to be found here, to the value of some thousand piasters.Here were several pounds of valuable Mumia materials from Persia, which is sold at three ducats. The Indian and American drugs

[57] Horn, pp. 176-179.

[58] See, for example: Costodia, p. 194, and in the exhaustive research of Farris & Storme.

come all from Spain and are chiefly given as presents. Here is prepared the Jerusalem Balsam, famous in these countries, which is a preparation made of all kinds of balsams and a number of aromaticks dissolved in spirit of wine. Of this they make yearly in the summer solstice a quantity that costs 150 ducats at Jerusalem. It is very useful in all fresh external wounds; but too hot to give internally. It is used in blood-spitting and contusions, from ten to twelve drops. The whole pharmacopoeia is valued at 100,000 piasters."[59]

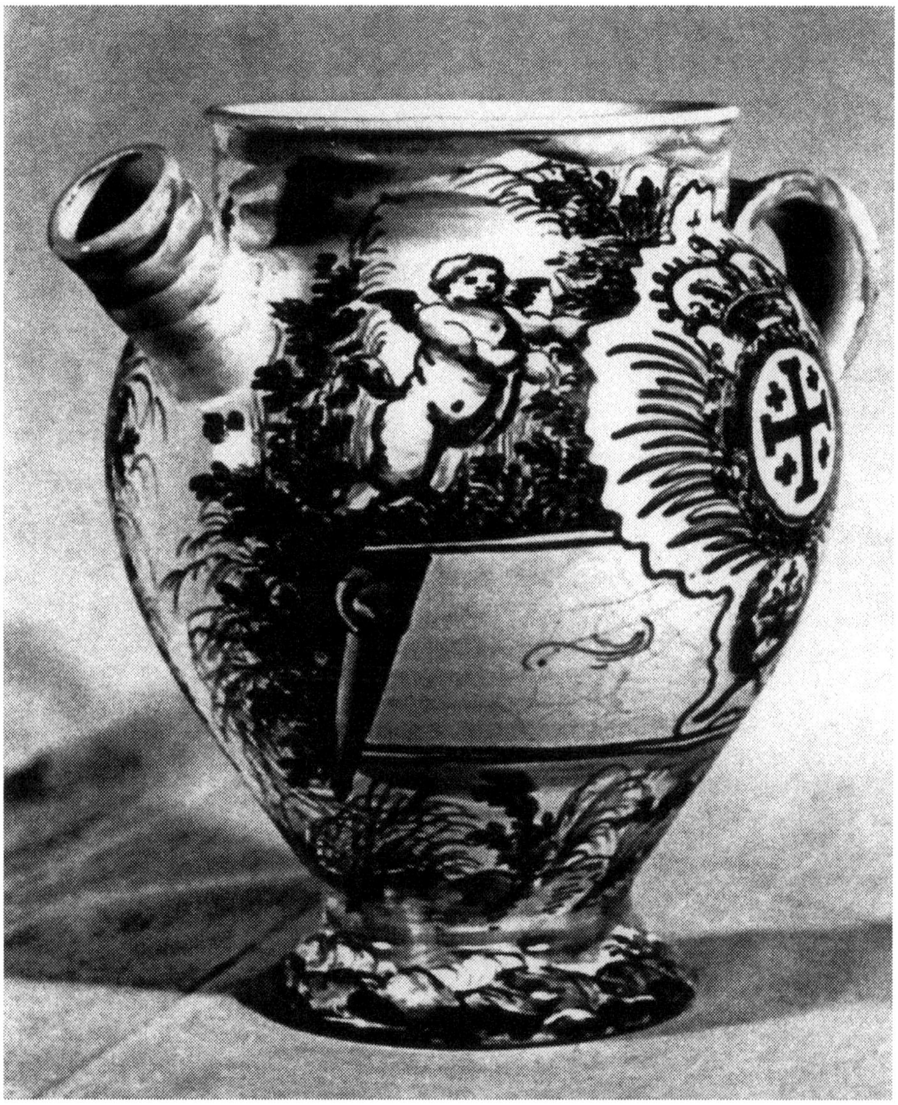

Figure 20: Ornamental vase sent to the Franciscan pharmacy in Jerusalem from the city of Savona in 1791.

The Jerusalem balsam was indeed considered one of the most famous medicines prepared in the Franciscan pharmacy. The inventor of this prestigious potion was Anthony Menzani of Cuna (1650-1729) a physician and pharmacist who was active in Jerusalem in the service of the monastery for forty-three years (1686-

[59] Hasselquist, p. 135.

1729). This personality is credited with the expansion of the institution, and it seems that in his lifetime the place also functioned as a hospital.[60] Many of those who used the Jerusalem balsam attested to its efficacy in curing disease and preventing epidemics. The use of Jerusalem balsam was also known in Acre, Beirut, and other remote places such as Constantinople and Palermo. The recipe for the Jerusalem balsam was a closely guarded secret and was concocted from plants that grew in the Jerusalem region or that could be obtained in Jerusalem. Among its dozens of ingredients were also spices used in the Temple incense, such as myrrh and frankincense, and medicinal drugs imported from Europe.[61] In the official archives of Venice, a description of the Jerusalem balsam has been reserved. It consists of forty ingredients that must be dissolved or melted in water and wine. When the wine evaporates, the rest of the materials stick like a kind of adhesive bandage on the wound and disinfect it.[62] According to Seetzen (1806) due to the lively demand for Jerusalem balsam, there were those who manufactured two kinds of counterfeit balsam which were cheaper. Besides the medicines they would import from Europe, the Franciscans would also prepare local medicines, some which came from a special garden of the monastery where they raised medicinal herbs.[63]

Private medicine

Many sick people preferred to use the services of private doctors. These physicians received their patients in private clinics, which were usually located in a shop. The clinic's equipment consisted of materia medica and utensils for various potions, a desk, rug, etc.[64] The shops that were used as clinics were owned generally by Muslims and were rented out for a period of a year or two. Thus for example there is mention in 1563 of a Jewish physician who rented a shop near the Chain Gate.[65] Some of the doctors who received wages from the imperial treasury for providing public medical service also engaged in private medical practice. One case is Kamil ben Mussa, a Jewish eye physician, whose private clinic was located in a shop in the al-'Attarin market which had formerly accommodated a Muslim physician.[66]

An example of a qualified physician who supported the Jewish Bikkur Holim institution and also engaged in private medicine was R. Refael Mordekhai Malki, although he did not practice privately for his livelihood. The story is told that when R. Yehuda Hahassid came to Jerusalem (1700) he, like many of his entourage, fell ill from the hardships of the trip. One of his companions recounts: "They sent for the expert physician who lived in Jerusalem, a Sephardic scholar, renowned in his knowledge of Torah and the art of medicine and prodigiously wealthy. That was the hakham R. Mordekhai Malki of blessed memory".

[60] Schittny, p. 44; Horn, p. 180.
[61] Bagatti, pp. 250-361.
[62] Schittny, pp. 43-44.
[63] Seetzen, pp. 205-206.
[64] Cohen, 16th Century, p. 269, no. 302.
[65] Cohen, Jewish, p. 211, fn. 189.
[66] Cohen, Jewish, p. 191.

R. Refael Malki arrived in the middle of the night to treat R. Yehuda Hahassid but was unable to be of help. From this account we also learn that Jews were forbidden to walk through the streets of the city at night, except in an emergency: "But in order to bring a physician to a sick person or a midwife to a laboring women, they are allowed to walk about throughout the night".[67] R. David de Silva, the grandson of R. Refael Mordekhai Malki, was a private physician. He makes no mention, not even indirectly, of the Bikkur Holim institution or the public hospital in Jerusalem. By his own account, he was called upon to treat many sick people of all of the religions in Jerusalem. Treatment was carried out in the patients' homes and in some instances, in his own house.[68]

Curing mental illness and magical medicine

Conventional medicine provided medical solutions for most of the diseases that were prevalent in Jerusalem and these generally satisfied the population. In contrast, mental illness and insanity were considered incurable, an attitude that was typical of the state of medicine throughout the world at that time. People who had lost their reason and thus either posed a risk to others or constituted a public nuisance were incarcerated until they recovered. This is actually not any kind of real treatment but rather a means of isolating them from society. One wing of the hospital that belonged to the waqf of al-Bimaristan al-Salahi handled the mentally ill.[69] The Jewish community had its own 'insane asylum' where the mentally ill were confined, and a tax was imposed by the government to maintain it.[70] Apparently other ethnic communities had their own versions of this institution.

Alongside of conventional medicine, there was widespread use of protective charms and medical amulets, and this recourse was acknowledged by physicians where they were unable to provide a cure using conventional techniques. Mental illness was an example of serious disease that in ancient times did not have any medical treatment that produced positive results. Consequently, and because of the severe symptoms that beset these patients, many people held the opinion that theirs was an unconventional illness that stemmed from demons and magical powers, and thus inevitably, only a magical cure could produce an appropriate medical solution. We find an example of this in the halachic treatise written by R. Nissim Hayim Mizrahi, rabbi of Jerusalem from 1745 (died in Jerusalem in 1749), in connection with a person who would periodically have fits of insanity; during an attack, they would chain him with iron shackles on his hands and feet in a closed room. Chaining the insane was the accepted treatment at that time in our region. Thus for example, in Damascus a Muslim traveler in 1184 notes this in his description of the hospitals in that city.[71] The rabbi was asked whether such a patient may be fed a chicken which had not been ritually slaughtered,

---

[67] Ya'ari, Travels, p. 328.
[68] P'ri Hadas, p. 52b, 133a-b, 139a.
[69] al-'Asali, Wata'iq, pp. 87-88; Ze'evi, p. 39.
[70] Cohen, 18th Century, pp. 318-319; Grayevsky, pp. 21,26.
[71] See: Ibn Jubayr, p. 283.

for some people attested that it was a proven cure: "Since such a cure is not a natural one as are the medicines prepared by the physicians, but rather because of its unique properties, the question is whether it is permitted or forbidden." At the end of an exhaustive halachic discussion, he ruled that curing an insane person this way was permitted.[72]

The very question shows that the rabbis were generally uncomfortable about the use of superstitions. Just how prevalent this phenomenon was can be seen in the fact that the by-laws of the Jewish community in Jerusalem from the middle of the sixteenth century refer to a "prohibition against making magical charms nor shall he order a gentile to do so, even for love".[73] This by-law implies that the gentiles did not hesitate to turn to the Jews and engage their services in making amulets. Using amulets and relics from holy sites in Jerusalem and the environs for medical purposes was also common among the pilgrims of all the religions.[74]

There were many charlatans in Jerusalem, and women "witches" especially became renowned. The physicians of the European school came out sharply against this phenomenon. R. Refael Mordekhai Malki also criticized it [75] as did his grandson, R. David de Silva who attacked these charlatans who had not received any medical training and yet called themselves "Doctor" with no justification. From de Silva, who was influenced by the eminent physician R. Tobias Cohen, we see that there was great tension and animosity between the genuine expert physicians who were duly trained and those who were charlatans.

> "The foolish do not know that a wise person can only be called such if he possesses wisdom and the dottore[76] can only use that title after achieving his doctorate, as is the practice in the Frankish cities. A person can only be called dottore after he has been qualified as a doctor, which is not what is done in these countries with their sycophancy, that even though a person has not a trace of Torah knowledge, he is called 'hakham' [rabbi] and the asodonico who knows little more than to let blood and make some kind of dressing, is called Signor Dottore. Thus they abet these corrupt charlatans, to boast and act arrogantly, to tyrannize the true hakham and physician. This includes the disgraceful phenomenon of the accursed loathsome old women who fall exhausted at night and during the day they go to seek out spells and incantations; they, too, are called doctors and sorcerers and Signorina Dottore by the gullible, and I am surprised to say, also by the wise – and the proof is that the latter rely on their opinion and take their cures. The reason for this is the magnitude of their folly and even if they do not know or understand any wisdom, they hate the wise doctor who has knowledge and intelligence, out of jealousy".[77]

---

[72] Mizrahi, chap. 6.
[73] Freiman, pp. 209, 213.
[74] Singer, p.202-203; Ya'ari, Igrot, 282.
[75] Malki, pp. 26-27.
[76] 'Dottore' is derived from the word 'dotto' meaning wise, learned.
[77] P'ri Hadas, p. 2a-b. Cf. Ma'aseh Tuviya, in the introduction to Part II (Sefer Eretz Hadasha), pp. 72-73.

These words of criticism were also directed to the patients themselves, some of them even from among the society of Torah scholars who used the services of the charlatans and thus gave legitimacy to this negative phenomenon. It appears that the phenomenon of trusting charlatans did not spare members of his own family. Thus, for example, when his sister-in-law's son was stricken by a disease that caused a contortion of his face, "the women began to use their charms as was their wont. They also said that it was the work of demons, and no physician's knowledge would avail here...I sent them a message that they should not follow these misguided ways and counsels for they are foolishness and vexation of the spirit which cannot know and understand; they walk in darkness." R. De Silva treated him by means of conventional medicine and cured him.[78] His approach was also expressed in his theoretical writings. In his book "P'ri Hadas" there is almost no mention of charms, amulets, or curing by using mystical methods ("practical kabbalah"). When he used the term 'סגולה' [variously 'charm' or 'special quality'] he used it in the sense of use or quality.[79]

In other words, despite the official disapproval of some of Jerusalem's rabbis,[80] many sought out charlatans who would offer them a variety of charlatan cures.[81] At the same time, it is worth noting that at that time, there was no definitive distinction between purely empirical medicine and magical medicine. In other words, there was a hazy and indeterminate area between medicines and charms. Such was the instance involving the milk of a female donkey (which presented a problem of dietary laws) cited by R. Moshe Hajiz, the son-in-law of R. Refael Mordekhai Malki:

> "The question of the milk of an unclean animal which is forbidden by the Torah...which can be used to cure one who is sick with dele azma[82] .This disease is confused with another one which is called apretiminto difigo which in Arabic is called dikitnefash[83] and people say that by using this charm they were cured, after drinking the milk of the female donkey for several days; I know from hearsay from my father-in-law R. Refael Mordekhai Malki that this disease poses a threat to life, and if the patient does not die today, then he will die the next day, and he is considered a person so ill that he is doomed to die of this disability. And now here in this case I consulted the physicians and they said that there was a danger and it is mentioned in the Book of Natural Cures also for people who spit up blood, who were cured by this method. Therefore, I call it a medicine that is guaranteed to work both by the

[78] P'ri Hadas, p. 133a-b

[79] Except for treatment of the evil eye, see; P'ri Hadas, p. 237a-b.

[80] See especially in the book by Menashe Sethune dedicated to uncompromising battle against the use of superstitious beliefs. He succeeded in rallying the support of all the rabbis of his day and even received the approval of all the rabbis of Jerusalem of all trends, see: Sethune, pp. 77-82.

[81] There are numerous accounts from the nineteenth century, see: Tobler, Medicine, pp. 2-10; Luncz, pp. 20-28; Halevi, pp. 362-368; Levi, History, pp. 19-24, and in the book by Nahamias on this subject.

[82] Asthma.

[83] Shortness of breath (dyspnea), in Arabic chik al-nafash.

physicians and by their books. Accordingly I have permitted the patient in this case to drink the milk about which he asked and let him drink as the physicians instructed..."[84]

Curing the sick of other religions

A physician in Jerusalem was not just physician to his co-religionists but rather served the entire population of the city. In this respect the profession of medicine must be said to cross religious and national boundaries. To demonstrate this consider the case where in January 1612 a physician at the Franciscan monastery was called out to treat a sick mufti who was visiting the area around the Temple Mount. He did this despite the fact that there was an absolute prohibition against non-Muslims entering this area, because at that time both of Jerusalem's regular physicians were absent, one of whom was a Muslim and the other, a Jew.[85]

The possibility of a physician practicing medicine regardless of his religious affiliation was reflected in the many accounts of physicians, both Jewish and Christian, who served in both public and private systems of medicine and their incorporation into the professional hierarchy. Despite this, a special sensitivity remained surrounding the treatment of Muslims by a Jew. Any failure or catastrophe that resulted from treatment by a Jew, a protected subject, could have aroused intemperate reactions towards the physician himself or towards the entire Jewish community.[86] R. David de Silva tells how he was called upon to treat an elderly Muslim merchant. The treatment involved blood-letting from the patient's wife and he was fearful that the patient would not survive the treatment and that he would be blamed for the merchant's death. This physician decided to hold a consultation of physicians, where he called in a group of physicians in order to hear their professional opinion and their consent to continue the treatment. Even though in this case he was protected by the Muslim law regarding accidents and claims, he preferred that the treatment be continued by another physician, presumably Muslim. And indeed, eventually it was proven that the method of treatment that he proposed was successful.[87] In light of this case, it is interesting to see a document of 1719 with a description of Yoseph the physician, a Jew who treated Muslims for altruistic reasons. Highly placed members within the Jewish community and outside it schemed against him and tried to collect illegal surcharges but he received protection against them by the qadi of Jerusalem.[88]

Jewish physicians offering treatment to patients of other religions occasionally raised halachic questions, for example, the use of foodstuffs forbidden by Jewish law in the preparation of various kinds of medicine. One

[84] Hajiz, I, chap. 290. Although the book was written by his father R. Ya'akov Hajiz, (1620-1674), he states here explicitly that he heard the law from his father-in-law, R. Refael Malki. It is quite certain that this happened in Jerusalem before 1693, before he left to go abroad. The use of donkey's milk for medicinal purposes is mentioned in Maimonides, Aphorisms, pp. 233, 244, 329. On the use of forbidden foods for medicinal purposes in Maimonides, see: Levinger, pp. 515-528.

[85] Boucher, p. 295.

[86] Cohen, Jewish, p. 189; Cohen, 18th Century, p. 323.

[87] P'ri Hadas, p. 62b.

[88] Cohen, 18th Century, p. 326, no. 280.

example of this is found in the treatise written by R. Nissim Hayim Mizrahi, the rabbi of Jerusalem from 1745: "Question: Regarding the practice of Jewish physicians who serve in the homes of officials who make medicinal preparations to which they add wine or honey made by gentiles and the like which are forbidden ...apparently the reason that this is forbidden is that he wants to do it is because he profits when he make medications from gentile's wine, for if he would make it of a permitted food, the physician would lose since honey made by Jews is sold expensively..."[89] From the question one can understand both that Jewish physicians treated the officials of the Ottoman government as well as the economic aspects that attended the preparation of medications. From his answer one may also learn of the important role of honey as a basic and vital ingredient in the preparation of medications:

> "I retract the reason I gave for physicians mixing the medication with honey; it is not for naught that they do this, as I had written, but rather it serves a specific purpose. The reason being that it is to neutralize the sharpness of the herbal medicines that must be administered to the patient for the cure which the sick person would be unable to eat, were it not for the honey which is mixed with the herbs so that the sick person can eat it. Therefore, the main taste enjoyment is from this honey".[90]

The Christians' attitude toward being treated by Jewish physicians in Jerusalem is somewhat different. The Franciscan friar Francesco Quaresmio who served in the land of Israel between 1616-1626 notes that it was forbidden for Franciscans in the land of Israel to obtain healing by a Jew except for unusual cases.[91] It seems that this was a Church regulation, periodically renewed, which stated that a Jew was forbidden to give treatment to Christian patients.

However, it is known that there were many places in Europe where this was not strictly enforced by the authorities, and members of the royal family and the priesthood availed themselves more than once of the services of Jewish physicians.[92] In Jerusalem, too, this directive was not observed and was not actually implemented. A chronicle of the Franciscans from 1625 tells of a judge in the city of Jerusalem who suggested a Syrian physician to the friars, but they contended that they had no use for such because they were already employing a Jewish physician. In spite of this, he charged them to pay the wages of the Syrian physician, 60 pennies monthly, even though the physician did not attend them.[93] Beyond the repressive policies of the local rule in Jerusalem one may learn from this case that the Jewish physician was able to pursue his vocation among the Christians without restraint, where his professional skill was the only criterion for evaluation. The practice of Jewish physicians treating Christian patients was apparently routine[94] and it

[89] Mizrahi, chapter 12, p. 29a.
[90] Mizrahi, chapter 12, p. 30a.
[91] Schur, Community, p. 376.
[92] Gelber, p. 348.
[93] Rozen, Ruins, p. 158.
[94] See, i.e. Cohen, 18th Century, p. 328, no. 285.

was patent that members of the Franciscan monastery preferred the ministering of a Jewish physician who came from Europe over other physicians, probably because of their superior level of professionalism and their shared cultural background. The Franciscan friar Horn tells how he used the services of a Jewish physician who had been trained at the University of Padua.[95]. R. David de Silva also used to treat Christians who requested his medical services thanks to the reputation he had acquired as an expert physician. In one case, he was called to treat a woman, apparently a nun, from the Armenian monastery in Jerusalem who was being strangled by a leech that attached itself to her throat. He extracted the leech by means of a piece of sponge attached to a long thread.[96]

Sanitary conditions in Jerusalem

The sanitation in Jerusalem and sanitary conditions during the Ottoman Period caused many infectious diseases and the outbreak of epidemics that exacted a heavy toll among the population.[97] This was the result of poor living conditions, overcrowding, and improper drainage that caused sewage to flow unchecked, and an overflow of refuse that collected in the city streets. Wild dogs also roamed the streets, which could not have contributed to public sanitation.[98]

Contemporary sources blamed the faulty health situation on several main causes: the Jerusalem climate, the food, and the drinking water. Rabbi Obadiah of Bertinoro at the end of the fifteenth century cites the climate as a factor:

> "And I must give thanks to God who until now has blessed me and I have not fallen ill as did all the other people who came here with me. Because most of the people who come to Jerusalem from distant lands fall ill because of the change in climate here and its constant fluctuations from hot to cold and from cold to hot. And all the winds in the world come and blow in Jerusalem."[99]

From his words one learns that many of the pilgrims and others who immigrated to the Land of Israel from Europe fell ill with colds, flu, and the like because of their inability to adjust to the local climate. Elzear Horn, as many of his contemporaries, ascribed the cause of the multiplicity of diseases in the Jerusalem area to the harsh climate, and among the common illnesses he lists: fever, ophtalmia, sciatica, dysentery, catarrh,

---

[95] Horn, pp. 179-180.

[96] P'ri Hadas, p. 139a.

[97] See: some figures in Arce, pp. 86-95; Hoade & Bagatti, in the introduction to Horn's book, p. 4; Singer, pp. 193, 198-199.

[98] In the Mamluk period, the rulers were strict about ridding the city of dogs, see: Drory, Emir, p. 198. The Italian traveler Alcarotti who visited Jerusalem in 1588 reports that the governor of the city gave instructions to kill the dogs infected with plague and bury them in the Jewish cemetery, see: Schur, Journey, p. 159; in early eighteenth century Jerusalem, the Jews were forced to remove the dogs killed by the Muslims, see: Ya'ari, Travels, pp. 362-363. Tobler, Medicine, p. 32 notes that "Rabies was not observed in Jerusalem, nor in other cities of the Orient".

[99] Ya'ari, Igrot, p. 137.

headaches, contagion, etc.[100] R. Refael Mordekhai Malki (at the end of the nineteenth century) describes the many types of fever that constituted the major chronic diseases in Jerusalem, but he ascribed the cause to the quality of food in Jerusalem:

> "I hereby inform the coming generations that most of the illnesses in Jerusalem are from excess moisture and a shortage of cooking due to the lack of natural warmth in the bodies. This all stems from the kinds of foods people are accustomed to eating both in summer and in winter, and they are cold foods with no spirituality in them, such as radishes and horseradish and squash and winter squash and watermelons… and let this be a rule to all generations: that all of the fruits and vegetables that Jerusalem and the land of Israel produce are colder and moister than all other countries and that is why those who fall sick are generally sick with fevers…."[101]

He also assigns great importance to the Jerusalem climate in effecting health: "The moisture in Jerusalem is not beneficial…although it helps the soil, it is harmful to the body, because the body is cured – by dryness."[102] In another place he adds: "…Therefore since the nature of water that we drink in the land of Israel is from wells, the water is drawn from the ground rather than flowing, and it is hard to digest and very heavy. It extinguishes natural heat and cancels out the attraction of the food from the stomach so that it cannot bear food, and even more so when the water is mixed with cold things, such as almond milk which is slippery like butter and milk and it is harmful to the intestines."[103] In fact, one of the real causes of the proliferation of disease in Jerusalem was the quality of the well water, except that Malki, true to his medical doctrine, ascribes the problem to the nature and temperament of the water and its effect on the body. It seems that the main problem with the drinking water in Jerusalem was the shortage of fresh water flowing within the city limits and wells that were not kept clean, forcing the residents of the city to drink foul well water. The well water also contained leeches and various kinds of reptiles.[104] The problem of water pollution was exacerbated particularly in the late summer. In a letter written by R. Avraham Gershon of Kitov in 1748 from Hebron, to his brother-in-law R. Yisrael Ba'al Shem Tov, he compares the fine quality of water in Hebron with the poor quality of the water in Jerusalem and Safad. For that reason, he did not fall ill but just to make sure, he asks for an "overall" amulet to protect him from disease.

> "Here (in Hebron) thank God there has not been any sickness, effecting even a fingernail. And the rabbis said to me, and they spoke truly, that all of the sick people in Jerusalem and Safad are stricken because they drink moldy water at the end of the summer. When the rain water reaches the bottom of the barrel, all of the dirt collects there, and when they scrub their roofs and courtyards, the water runs

---

[100] Horn, p. 178.
[101] Malki, pp. 58-59.
[102] Malki, p. 77.
[103] Malki, p. 60.
[104] P'ri Hadas, p. 139a; P'ri Hadash commentary on Yoreh Deah, 84, subpar. 9.

into the well. Then when they drink the well water, they drink all of the filth, and they are stricken – but in Hebron they drink water from the wells of our father Abraham, Isaac, and Jacob who dug wells of good, healthful water. There is never any disease in them, except by Divine decree, and a plague has been brought here from other places that lasted twelve years, God protect us. If you would send me a comprehensive type of amulet so that I would not need a new one every year, how good that would be and would bring me great satisfaction."[105]

The public baths

The only practical solution for personal hygiene was the public baths. An increase in the population of the city in the middle of the sixteenth century led to the construction and renovation of the bathhouses.[106] In the middle of the seventeenth century there were six public baths in Jerusalem: Hammam al-Battrak, Hammam Seti Miriam, Hammam al-Sultan, Hammam al-'Eain, Hammam al-Giammal, and Hammam al-Shifa.[107] Most of these had been operating in the Mamluk Period and even before that.[108] Renowned in particular was the Hammam al-Shifa which means the medicinal bath, since those who bathed there believed that its waters provided a curative for their afflictions, apparently based on the tradition that the source of its waters was the Siloam Spring which was known for its therapeutic qualities.[109] This bath is mentioned in 1677 by R. Moshe ben Habib, one of the rabbis of Jerusalem: "There is a bath close to the Temple Mount, the site of the Holy Temple, and it is called in Arabic 'Hammam al-Shifa' and they say that its waters come from the top of this spring (the Siloam)."[110]

The institution of the public bath provided service to all of Jerusalem's residents, although the Muslims who lived in the city enjoyed preferential treatment. The supervisor of the markets (muhtesib) had to check daily that the water was clean and to make sure that there were different towels for the Muslims and for the other protected subjects and the peasants.[111] Entry to the bath entailed payment of a fee for the bath, a towel, and cleaning of the body, as told by R. Gedalya of Siemiatycze in the beginning of the eighteenth century:

"The public bath of Jerusalem is very splendid and has many rooms, all of them warm. There is warm and there is warmer, and each person sits where he wishes, even a Jew. The cost of the bath is one coin...and also for the servant who gives a robe for the bather to put on in front for the sake of

[105] Ya'ari, Igrot, 282.
[106] Cohen, Jewish, p. 220.
[107] Horn, p. 211; Singer, p. 197.
[108] The Hammam al-Battrak was already in operation during the Crusader Period, see: Patrich, Structure, p. 12; Frenkel, Establishment, p. 32.
[109] On the medicinal qualities of the waters of Siloam, see: Amar, Metamorphosis, pp. 214-217.
[110] Ben-Habib, chap. 128. This bath house is also known in our times, and is located at the end of the street of the shops near the gate leading to the Temple Mount.
[111] Cohen, 16th Century, pp. 144-145, doc. 137, fn. 1; p. 146, doc. 141. Horn, p. 214 notes that in the Hammam al-Giammal was used only rarely, due to the poor sanitary conditions prevailing there.

modesty, one must pay a coin and for the servant who bathes the person and washes him, also the same amount."[112]

A visit to the public bath was considered a necessary practice in 18th century Jerusalem and was included among the basic necessities that the husband was obliged to pay to his divorced wife. In fact, he had to pay for all of the woman's hygienic requirements; besides entry to the baths, he also had to pay for her soap and laundering her clothes.[113]

The standard of medicine in Jerusalem

The end of the sixteenth century already began to witness the decline of the Ottoman Empire. This process also effected the standard of medicine in the land of Israel. Thus, too, the improvement of the water supply to the city by Sultan Suleiman the Magnificent must be seen as a short-lived episode which was not typical of the policy of most of the Ottoman rulers. It may be generally stated that the period of Ottoman rule did not bring any substantial change to the inferior standard of medicine in the country. This was reflected in two major areas: the system of medical education and the maintenance of a proper health system. The medical technique practiced in the country was in fact a continuation of the ancient Hippocractic-Galenian system which was adopted and refined by Muslim medical science in the Middle Ages [Fig. 21]. During this period it was hard to find in this region important centers which boasted scholars of stature. In that sense one may consider the encyclopedia of Daud al-Antaki of the sixteenth century (d. 1599) the swan song of classical medieval medical literature. Al-Antaki studied medicine under other physicians in Cairo and Damascus, using the traditional method accepted in the Middle Ages.[114] There is scant information about western medicine in his book.[115] He does mention Jerusalem several times as a source of medicine, but it is clear that most of his information reflects classical medicine, and a considerable part of this information is borrowed from even earlier sources.

The land of Israel under the Ottoman Empire, like under the Mamluks, was considered a backwater which provided little of interest to the ruler. Due to its remote location from the centers of culture and administration, physicians of any prominence avoided settling there. That is apparently the reason for the incentives granted by the authorities to physicians who were sent to serve in Jerusalem. In the beginning of the sixteenth century one may perceive the desire of the authorities to maintain a proper system of public health in Jerusalem which ensured inter alia an efficient system of supervision and enforcement. For example, they ensured that there would be a number of qualified physicians in Jerusalem on a regular

[112] Ya'ari, Travels, p. 359.
[113] Cohen, 18th Century, doc. 445, p. 466; doc. 450, p. 469.
[114] al-Muhibbi, II, pp. 141-142.
[115] Plessner, p. 139.

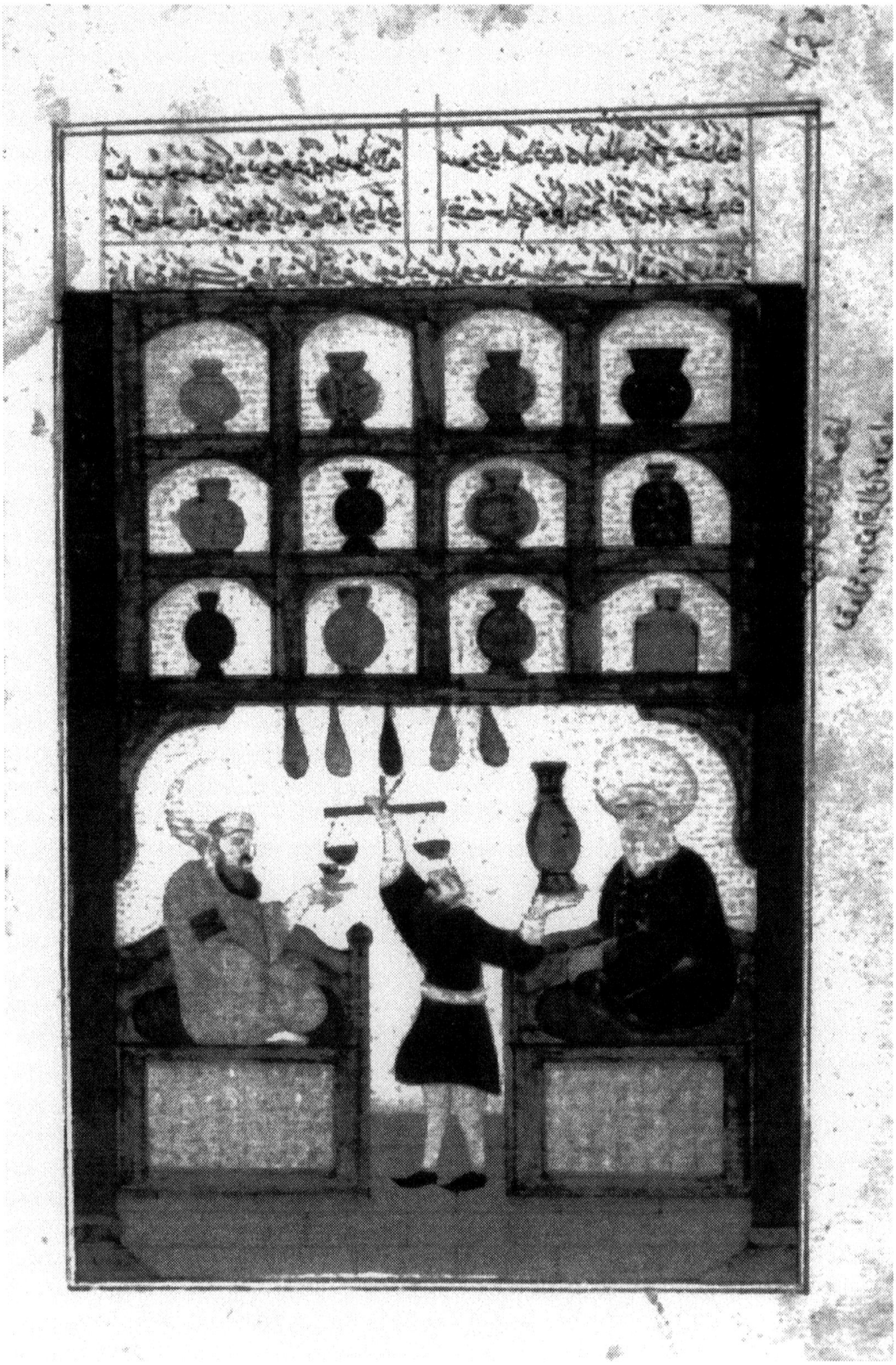

Figure 21: Segment of an Ottoman illuminated manuscript (1781) from the medical treatise of Ibn Sina. Most medical treatises that were used in the Ottoman Empire belonged to the genre of Galenic-Arabic medicine.

basis. The government's involvement in maintaining the medical system with proper operating procedures undoubtedly contributed to the fact that Jerusalem had physicians of a high professional standard. As will be seen later on, beginning in the seventeenth century, one may discern an erosion in the high standards and institutions of medicine in Jerusalem.

In any event, medicine was considered a distinguished and essential profession, and those engaged in it belonged to an elite social and economic class. The Jewish physicians, rabbinical and Karaite alike, earned a reputation as professional practitioners. There are many accounts of this in Christian and Muslim sources which cannot be considered suspect. The traveler Rauwolf (circa 1573) praises the Jewish physicians, incidental to a description of the Jews of Jerusalem.[116] The Franciscan friar Eugene Roger who served in the land of Israel from approximately 1628-1635 cites among the professions of Jews of Jerusalem – physicians, who were among its scholars.[117] Elzear Horn who described with wonderment the institutions of Franciscan medicine in Jerusalem noted in the same breath that in 1729 he preferred to use the services of an Ashkenazic Jewish physician who lived in Jerusalem.[118] This may be attributed to the fact that they came from the same place of origin and that he preferred a physician who represented the European, modern school of thought in medicine.

Furthermore, the expert Jewish physicians were acknowledged as authorities by the central government and by their Muslim colleagues. When the "Head of the physicians" was compelled to absent himself from Jerusalem, Jewish and Christian physicians could take his place. Moreover, they could advance professionally to the highest position, even to be the "Head of the physicians" in Jerusalem, at least temporarily.[119] In contrast with the sources that laud the high standards of the Jerusalem physicians, R. Refael Mordekhai Malki presents an opposite picture. According to him there were no qualified physicians in Jerusalem at all:

"And if there is a physician in Jerusalem, he is not an expert,. There are many physicians who are neither expert nor learned, and there are none who are both expert and learned. The reason is that all over the Orient and the lands of Turkey and the West do not know the methods and laws of medicine ...[120] From this we may see and know why it is impossible for a physician in Jerusalem, because its residents and scholars do not recognize genuine medicine and its ways. In their eyes, anyone claiming to be a physician and the true physician are equal...[121] In the end: as the situation of Jerusalem stands today and the physicians in it, one is not allowed to use physicians at all, and anyone who acts as they instruct is risking human life...so that when

[116] Schur, Community, p. 364.
[117] Roger, p. 370.
[118] Horn, pp. 179-180.
[119] Cohen, Jewish, pp. 189-190.
[120] Malki, p. 68.
[121] Malki, p. 72.

I see this glorious city, (may it be rebuilt speedily) which has no hope of having a physician and also when we see the danger that these derelict physicians cause to the sick, I will express my opinion of them and I will advise the coming generations who live here as well as in all the cities of Turkey and the West that with these physicians who live among them, they would be better off if there were none rather than having theire injurious presence. Let them leave the sick in the hand of the Almighty who is the true healer and who safeguards the gullible, rather than hand over the sick to these."[122]

The harsh criticism that R. Refael Malki had of Jerusalem's physicians is not directed exclusively at the Jewish physicians but rather at the poor standards of the profession in general. The sources cited here indicate that R. Refael Malki is reflecting the reality of the Jerusalem of his time, namely the last third of the seventeenth century, rather than an earlier state. R. Refael is plainly describing a reality where local medicine is at its nadir. This is undoubtedly the result of the process of decline and deterioration that characterized the land of Israel at that time. With the weakening of the central government and the absence of proper and orderly administration, the efficiency and standards of local medicine were also eroded. R. Refael Malki's criticism indicates that in his time there was none too strict an insistence on the professional standards of physicians in Jerusalem. Some studied the art of medicine theoretically without ever delving deeply; some only studied under other physicians without becoming familiar with the professional literature, and some even declared themselves physicians without ever serving under or interning under another physician, which constituted in some cases a death penalty for their patients.[123] This situation reflects the lack of professional supervision or high standards which had characterized medicine in the beginning of the Ottoman Period. While the records of Muslim courts in the eighteenth century reveal many legal deliberations involving compensation for medical negligence, [124] these were deliberations revolving around the criminal aspect. At that same time, there is no evidence of any sincere desire or ability on the part of the authorities to preserve binding professional standards, for apparently those who headed the professional hierarchy (the Head of the physicians) were themselves not of the highest standard. R. Refael Malki's criticism must also be viewed against a backdrop of the development of modern medicine in Europe. As a physician who had studied in Europe, he regarded himself a genuine expert physician representing the pinnacle of advanced medicine and the local physicians, as backward and ignorant. This was not just criticism of their professional standards but also of the proper arrangements for supervision and administration, for the physicians who had been trained in institutions in Europe were subject to a death penalty if they did not faithfully perform their duties.[125]

[122] Malki, p. 73.
[123] Malki, p. 71.
[124] Cohen, 18th Century, pp. 323-330.
[125] Malki, pp. 28-29, 71.

R. Refael Malki's words express a revolutionary process that was taking place in Europe's universities of note, which took the form of abandoning the old Galenian theoretical study in favor of a new empirical scientific method based on observation and practical experiments. At the same time, there was a significant development in the fields of anatomy and chemistry. The academic curricula stressed the study of botany according to the new literary genre created by the herbalists of that time. This literature includes illustrated plant guides, with a large variety of plants beyond those brought by Dioscorides in De Materia Medica. In this field, university-sponsored botanical gardens were established to house plants from all over the globe, including medicinal plants from the New World.[126]

R. Refael Malki's words correspond to the description given by Volney who visited the land of Israel around the year 1785. Volney painted a bleak portrait of the status of medicine in the Syria and Egypt of his time. Although his words seem a bit extreme, he was apparently not far from the truth:

> "The intimate connection between the arts and sciences, leaves no room to doubt that the latter are still more neglected, or to confess the truth, totally unknown. The barbarism of Syria, as well as that of Egypt, is compleat; and from the familiarity which is usually found in the different provinces of the same empire, we may form the like judgment of all the countries under the dominion of the Turks. In vain have some persons denied this assertion; in vain do they talk of *colleges, places of education, and books*; these words in Turkey convey not the same ideas as with us. The age of the Califs is past among the Arabs, and yet to begin among the Turks. These two nations have at present neither geometricians, astronomers, musicians, nor physicians. Scarcely can we meet with one of the latter who knows how to bleed with a fleam; when they have ordered a cautery, applied fire, or prescribed some common recipe, their knowledge is exhausted; and consequently the valet de chambre of an European is consulted as an Esculapius; where indeed should physicians be formed, since there are no establishments of the kind?"[127]

The influence of western medicine on Muslim medicine begins to show results in the seventeenth century. This is expressed, for example, in the Muslim medical literature, in references to new western medications and the translation of western medical treatises.[128] However, the effect on the overall Muslim medical system was minimal, and even then was limited to the larger, more important centers in the Ottoman Empire, in Constantinople, Aleppo, Cairo, and the like, and to Jerusalem which was considered a backwater. Typical of this is a medical book copied by the hakham Moshe Halevi al-qudsi (=of Jerusalem), a Karaite copyist who was active in the land of Israel and Egypt in the sixteenth and seventeenth centuries. The book was called

[126] Ruderman, pp. 107-108; Palmer, pp. 100-117.
[127] Volney, II, p. 443.
[128] Issacs, pp. 52-57.

"What Every Physician Must Know".[129] This was actually an abridged version of the treatise by Ibn al-Baytar (d. 1248), who was active in this region during the Ayyubid period and it does not contain any significantly new information. Another example is the collection of manuscripts preserved by the Greek Patriarch in Jerusalem including thirteen documents dealing with medicine from the sixteenth to the nineteenth centuries.[130] The very fact that they are written in Greek rather than in Latin or Arabic (except for one manuscript from 1708 written in Arabic) or in other European languages is evidence that this is the product of copying and a theoretical study of classical medical texts rather than the actual practice of medicine, and certainly not the study of modern medicine which originated at the European academies. In any event, the "new scientific" medicine was unknown throughout the Ottoman Empire in the eighteenth century and began to really be a force only in the last quarter of the nineteenth century.[131] Another factor that contributed to the introduction of western medicine into the Orient were non-Muslim physicians who received their training in Europe and visited the East. Some of them even lived for extended periods in this area.[132] The foreign physicians were warmly welcomed by the government, due to the shortage of skilled Ottoman physicians.[133] Especially noteworthy is the migration of many Jewish physicians from Spain, Portugal, and Italy to the Ottoman Empire, particularly to Constantinople. Many of them had studied at the Christian universities of Europe, such as Padua and Pisa, and brought with them extensive knowledge of both eastern and western medical science. The Jewish physicians were incorporated into the imperial service and some earned the privilege of an appointment as personal physician to the various sultans. The Ottoman administration records show that the medical profession was dominated by Jews. The number of Jewish physicians was greater than that of Muslim and Christian physicians, relative to their ratio in the population.[134] Greater importance must be attributed to this factor, when examining the question of how to date the introduction of modern Western medicine into Jerusalem in particular and the land of Israel in general during the Ottoman Period.

Materia medica

During the Ottoman Period a wide variety of materia medica was in use in Jerusalem, of vegetable, animal, and mineral origin. Some of the medicinal drugs were local while some were imported from distant countries. The most important source for learning about materia medica is the book "P'ri Hadas" written by R. David de Silva, who dedicates an entire chapter entitled "P'ri Megaddim(=choice fruit)".[135] This section contains some two hundred entries with a description of various foods and medicines. The treatise written by

[129] Gamil, p. 555.
[130] Clark, pp. 6-8, 397-398.
[131] Murphey, pp. 379, 397-398.
[132] Isaacs, p. 56.
[133] Murphey, p. 384.
[134] Heyd, Moses, pp. 152-170; Lewis, pp. 223-234.
[135] P'ri Hadas, p. 37a-45b.

his grandfather, R. Refael Mordekhai Malkhi, also mentions many materia medica.[136] Another important source of information is brought by Swiss physician and scientist Titus Tobler in the description of his visit to the city in 1845. Tobler describes at length the condition of medicine and medical institutions in Jerusalem, in an age where modern medicine had not yet succeeded in leaving its imprint. His description furnishes an accurate portrayal of the state of medicine and an unusual documentation of the traditional medicine which was still being practiced in the city. Part of his description includes a comprehensive list of the materia medica as he meticulously recorded them on his visit to the spice market (Suq al- 'Attarin) in one of the shops selling folk medicines.[137]

An analysis of the list of materials mentioned by R. David de Silva and Tobler shows a strong similarity as to the source of the materials and their proportional distribution. This is also true of a comparison of the composition of historical lists from earlier periods: for example, lists of materia medica taken from the writings of Hippocrates, Dioscorides, and later essays from the Middle Ages on the one hand, and modern lists drawn up at shops selling medicines in Israel on the other.[138] These results are summarized in **Table 3** :

Table no. 3

Some materia medica in use in Jerusalem in the 18th-19th centuries according to R. David de Silva and Tobler, compared with other lists

Source	RDS in Pri Megaddim	%	Tobler	%	Medieval	%	Modern Israel	%
Vegetable	124	67.5	60	74	190	85.9	264	85
Animal	32	17.5	7	8.7	9	4.1	20	6.6
Mineral	13	7	10	12.4	15	6.8	19	6.1
Other	15	8	4	4.9	7	3.2	2.3	6
Total	184	100	81	100	221	100	310	100

These figures show that the overwhelming majority of drugs used either separately as a medicine or as an ingredient in complex medicines are of vegetable origin, while only a few come from an animal, mineral, or other source. It should be noted that these are not precise statistical figures, but the data brought here does not significantly alter the general picture presented. Furthermore, the number of materia medica in use in

[136] E.g., Malki, pp. 62-67, 77-79.
[137] Amar & Lev, Tobler, pp. 604-607.
[138] Amar & Lev, Survey, pp. 16-17.

Jerusalem at that time was actually greater. Thus, for example, we find mention of additional materia medica in the writings of travelers[139] and in the records of the Muslim courts in Jerusalem.[140]

One of the most interesting facts appearing in contemporary sources are references to new edible and medicinal plants that spread through Europe and the East following the discovery of America. Some of these plants were introduced to the world of traditional medicine and even reached Jerusalem, and thus we are made aware of the first signs of a pharmacological impact on the city from the West. These plants appear in **Table no. 4:**

Table no. 4: Edible and medicinal plants from the New World

Plant	RDS	Tobler	Tobias Cohen
Ipecac (Cephaelis ipecacuanha)		+	
Guaiac (Guaiacum sanctum)	+		+
Tabacco (Nicotiana tabacum)	+	+	+
Quinine (Cinchona sp.)	+	+	+
Soapwort (Sassafras officinale)	+	+	+
Sarsaparilla (Smilax sp.)		+	+
Cacao (Theobroma cacao)	+		+

The burgeoning of European medicine in Ottoman Jerusalem

The quality of Jewish physicians in Jerusalem in the sixteenth and middle of the seventeenth centuries was high, at least in comparison with the Muslim and Christian physicians. Therefore, it would not be an exaggeration to credit the initial introduction of European medicine into Jerusalem to the Jewish physicians, and in considerable measure to the earlier policy of the Ottoman Empire. The Ottoman administration brought about a change in status to the Jewish community in Jerusalem, which also had an indirect effect on improving the level of medicine in Jerusalem. The growth of the Jewish community, the product of mass

139 E.g., Horn, p. 180.

140 E.g., Cohen, 18th Century, pp. 324-325, no. 279.

migration form Europe, was a decisive factor in the cultural character of the Jewish community, and it indirectly influenced the Jewish community throughout the land of Israel.

A list of Jewish physicians of Jerusalem in the sixteenth- eighteenth centuries shows that approximately one quarter of them came from various European centers; Poland, the Iberian peninsula, and Italy. Though it is only a partial list, it is enough to reveal some characteristic features. It seems that in most cases the physician mentioned was retired, that is, someone who had undergone official medical training but did not actually practice medicine while in Jerusalem. The fact that these physicians came to Jerusalem (which was considered part of the hinterland of the Ottoman Empire) was because of the central role that Jerusalem, together with Safad, played in spiritual life. These Jews would come to study the Torah and Kabbalah, not to practice medicine; nonetheless, this had an impact on the nature of medicine in Jerusalem.

The Jewish physicians coming from Europe were a link and a mediating force in the contact between eastern and western culture and were in effect harbingers of the burgeoning of modern Western medicine in the land of Israel. This does not mean only the physicians themselves but also the new population that preferred treatment by the conventional medical techniques of their country of origin. Specially noteworthy is the large influx of Jews to the land of Israel, who also came to Jerusalem from the Iberian peninsula and from Italy.[141] Throughout the Ottoman Period, close ties were maintained between the rabbis of the land of Israel and those in Italy, a connection that was also reflected in donations, influences in the Torah world, and in leadership of the community where Italian Jews served.[142] The uninterrupted connection between Jerusalem and Italy undoubtedly influenced the introduction of the European medical school of thought into the land of Israel. Furthermore, most of the Jews who studied medicine in Europe and lived in Jerusalem were trained in Italy, particularly at the University of Padua. At that time Italian hospitals were considered the most advanced in all of Europe.

The advent of European medicine to the land of Israel was expressed in medical literature written or used by the Jewish physicians, who had come from Europe, during their stay in the land of Israel, Thus, for example, in the medical treatises of R. Hayyim Vital, Tobias Cohen, R. Refael Malki, and R. David de Silva, we find that a considerable part of the names of the medicines and diseases appear in foreign languages, in Spanish, Portuguese, Italian, and Latin, occasionally spiced with Arabic or Turkish.[143] These physicians used terminology in European languages during their practical work as well. Nonetheless it must be observed that most of the materia medica that they mention are still part of the inventory of traditional medicine and only a small share represent medicines from the New World. Horn, for example cites in his medical treatise the precise prescription written for him in Latin-Italian by the Jewish physician who was called to the Franciscan

[141] David, Immigration, pp. 112-121.
[142] Shulvass, pp. 68-73, 84-88; Benayahu, Anthology, pp. 55-66.
[143] See comment by Rivlin, Collection, II, pp. 7-8, fn. 6.

hospital to treat him.[144] This prescription, incidentally, shows that Horn suffered from hemorrhoids and the treatment consisted of dosing with various laxative preparations, among them "one purge with six drachmas of Cassia, Cathaliconis (its name in Portuguese; medicinal rhubarb – Rheum officinalis) and a potion made of almond milk, honey, and roses (orzato con mel rosato)". These medications were popular among the Jewish community in Jerusalem.[145]

Another factor that contributed to the introduction of European medicine in Jerusalem was the Franciscan pharmacy in Jerusalem which was considered the largest in the Near East [Fig. 22]. Evidence of this was the variety of medications from all over the world that were available there, a staff of certified pharmacists trained in Europe, and modern medical equipment. Since there was no other pharmacy in Jerusalem, it served people of all Christian denominations and distributed medicine free of charge [Fig. 23].[146] The monastery also had at its disposal a library rich in professional medical literature of the European school.[147] This institution is known already from the beginning of the seventeenth century but due to the restrictions imposed by the Ottoman administration, operated on a limited basis. In fact it was only during the eighteenth century that it was expanded and developed, and its influence on the character of medicine in Jerusalem is felt relatively later. One example of a medication that originated in the New World that was introduced into use by the Franciscans is quinine (Cinchona). Horn, in the first half of the eighteenth century, notes that quinine (which he refers to as 'China-China') is used for cases of malaria and had proven its efficacy.[148] R. David de Silva also attested that he had used it: "China-China ...I tried it because it is good for all types of fever and catarrh and for all kinds of the cold diseases".[149] There are more examples of new materia medica in Jerusalem but the overwhelming majority of medications sold in Jerusalem in the mid nineteenth century are still defined as traditional medical substances.[150] A brief prologue of modern European medicine in the land of Israel can also be seen in the activity of the military doctors in Napoleon's army which invaded the country in 1799. They applied new techniques in medicine in general and military medicine in particular but this had no effect on the state of medicine in Jerusalem.[151]

In effect even the Jewish physicians who came from Europe did not succeed in making a significant change in the status of medicine in the land of Israel (and throughout the Ottoman Empire). Their influence was limited to the holy cities, particularly Jerusalem and Safad where many new arrivals congregated, some of whom were educated and belonged to the elite classes. Nonetheless, in the large Jewish centers the medical system was still dominated by Eastern medicine. This is in addition to the practice of medicine through

[144] Horn, p. 180.
[145] Cf: Malki, pp. 45, 62-64; Cohen, 18th Century, p. 324, no. 279.
[146] Horn, pp. 176-178.
[147] See in introduction to Horn, pp. 6-7.
[148] Horn, p. 181.
[149] P'ri Hadas, p. 44b.
[150] Tobler, Medicine, pp. 15-16.
[151] Levi, History, pp. 12-18.

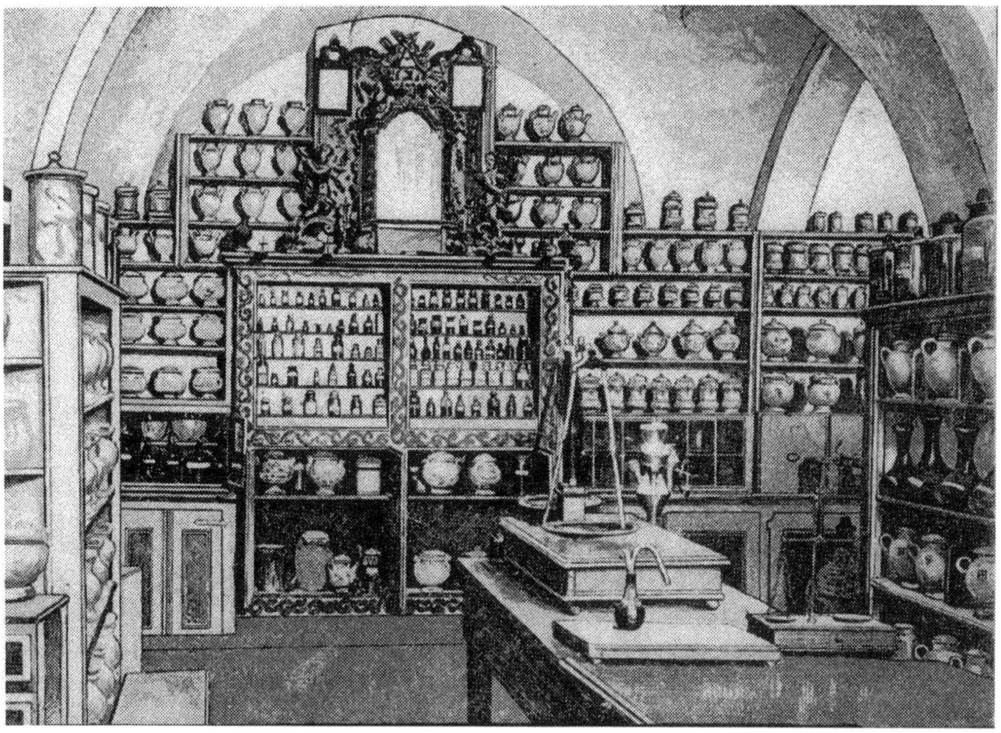

Figure 22: The Franciscan pharmacy in Jerusalem (nineteenth century print).

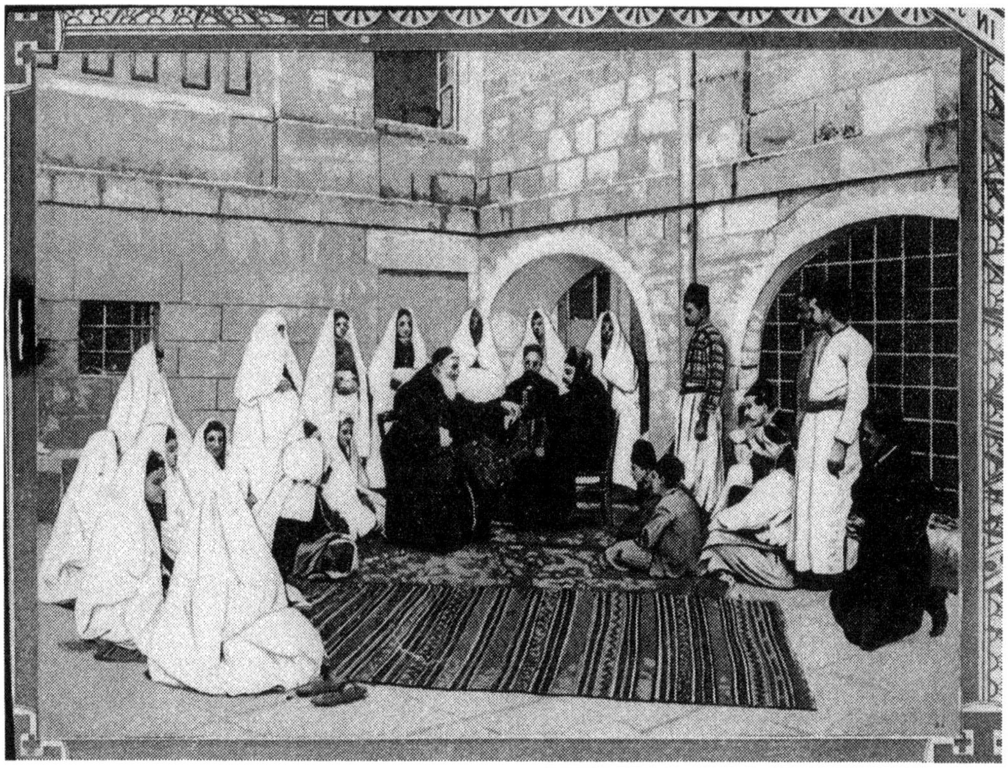

Figure 23: Medical treatment administered at the Franciscan pharmacy in Jerusalem (early twentieth century).

magic, which was a well developed industry in Jerusalem. It would seem that the phenomenon of the Jewish European physicians in Jerusalem and the effect of the school of European medicine, particularly Italian, was insignificant. It was one of the off-shoots of the more central phenomenon – the development of important centers of Torah and Kabbalah in the land of Israel and the importance of Jerusalem as a holy city. These physicians were not able to significantly influence the poor level of medicine in Jerusalem in the seventeenth and eighteenth centuries, and in this sense, they were before their time. Moreover, an analysis of the medical writings left by prominent physicians of the European school who were active in Jerusalem, such as Tobias Cohen, R. Refael Mordekhai Malki, and R. David de Silva shows that the school of medicine practiced by them was still based on the principles of the traditional Galenian-Arabic system. Thus, these physicians represent a transition stage between ancient and modern medicine.

It seems that only from the middle of the nineteenth century onward can one feel the effect of modern medicine in the land of Israel in any meaningful way.[152] It is only from this period onward that we find hospitals that focus on medical treatment rather than a complex of social welfare activities, as was accepted practice in earlier times. The revised purpose and functioning of the hospital began in Europe in the sixteenth and seventeenth centuries[153] but in Jerusalem it began only later, during the nineteenth century.

[152] Reiss, p. 3.
[153] Seidler, pp. 19-21.

Epilogue
The beginnings of modern medicine in Jerusalem

The information and studies that have been written about medicine in Jerusalem in the nineteenth and twentieth centuries are abundant and deserve a separate summary essay on the subject. I would like to present here at the end of the book a brief review of some of the milestones in the development of modern medicine in Jerusalem and a short bibliographical list for those who wish to learn more.

Over the course of the nineteenth century, which marks a transition from the medieval ages to the modern age, medicine in Jerusalem underwent significant changes. Part of this process is connected to the decline and fall of the Ottoman Empire, a consequence of the involvement of Europe in events in the land of Israel. The European powers in their quest for a political foothold and diplomatic influence encouraged, among others, the establishment of philanthropic institutions and even offered their financial support. This is the backdrop for the revitalized interest in the land of Israel by scholars, researchers, and travelers on the one hand, and religious elements on the other, which wished to be benefactors to the inhabitants of Jerusalem . It is during this period that we witness the founding of modern hospitals and the arrival of certified physicians trained in the modern medical techniques practiced in Europe.

Jewish institutions of healing

The research reflects a controversy as to who must be credited with the beginning of the age of modern medicine and pharmacology and the question of who built the first Jewish hospital. There is no doubt that the Christian Mission had a decisive role in the advancement and acceleration of this process. In 1838 the Dutch Association of Missionaries dispatched to Jerusalem two Jews who had converted to Christianity; one a physician by the name of Gertsmann and the second, the pharmacist Bergheim. They established a hospital on Mount Zion that also was active in the propagation of Christianity. For lack of a modern hospital in the city, the Jews were forced to use the Mission's services, despite the objections of Jerusalem's rabbis. In response to this dilemma, Dr. Ludwig Philippson promoted the idea of building a Jewish hospital in Jerusalem which won the support of Montefiore and Rothschild. However, the idea of attaching to the hospital a school in the spirit of the Enlightenment kindled the opposition of many groups, and his plan ultimately failed. The problem raised by medicine as practiced at the mission led the leaders of the community to appeal to Moses Montefiore, who had in the meantime sent Dr. Simon Fraenkel to Jerusalem in 1843 to open a clinic that would treat patients free of charge. Montefiore provided funds for the salary of Fraenkel (who served at his post until 1858), the establishment of a pharmacy, and all of the expenses of the clinic and its equipment, which operated for some twenty years.

The first serious attempt to supply a solution to the missionary activity was the building of the first Jewish hospital in 1844, at the initiative of the Sephardic Community, and it managed to operate for four years. A few years later, one Dr. Bernard Neumann, a Jewish physician, was invited by the House of Rothschild to establish a Jewish hospital, in 1854. This hospital (named after Meyer Anshel Rothschild) also provided medical services to Muslims and Christians. The pharmacy was directed by Dr. Moshe Robovitz who immigrated to Jerusalem in 1854, and there are some who credit him with being the first Jewish pharmacist in Jerusalem.

Later on additional hospitals were established: Bikkur Holim and Misgav La-Dakh which operated on a more limited scale, in several rented rooms. The Bikkur Holim Hospital was founded by public activists from the separatists circa 1867, and funded by the *haluka* moneys and contributions collected abroad for this purpose. This was the culmination of an extended period undergone by the "Bikkur Holim of the Separatists" which had been established in the first third of the nineteenth century until Bikkur Holim began operations as a modern medical institution (the hospital moved to its new building in Strauss Street in 1925). The Misgav La-Dakh Hospital was founded by well-to-do Sephardic Jews in 1879. In 1876 a clinic was also opened in Jerusalem in the style of the modern health fund clinics. The founder of the clinic was Dr. Shraga Feivel Pufeles, who worked with funding from Holland. He had previously worked as a physician on the staff at Bikkur Holim. In 1896 the Ezrat Nashim Clalit Association established a small hospital for mentally ill and terminally ill patients, which was located at the entrance to the Old City. In 1904 it moved to its new location and was called the "Yesha Aharon" Hospital. These institutions of healing could not provide for all of the needs of the growing population of Jerusalem. Relief came with the opening of new hospitals outside the walls of the Old City: Rothschild Hospital (1888), Sha'arei Tzedek Hospital (1902), and Bikkur Holim (1910). One of the signs of the times also was the initiation of private clinics, modern pharmacies, and government supervision against pharmacists who were not licensed.

One of the most prevalent types of disease in Jerusalem was eye disease. There was an attempt to establish a Jewish hospital for eye diseases in 1900 but it closed after one year. Another hospital worthy of note was the hospital for eye diseases that was founded in 1908 and later became renowned, thanks to its director Dr. Avraham (Albert) Ticho who succeeded in dramatically reducing the incidence of Trachoma which was widespread among the population of Jerusalem and the environs.

There are also accounts of dentistry in Jerusalem at the end of the nineteenth and beginning of the twentieth century. In 1913 two registered nurses arrived in Jerusalem from America, who had been sent by the Zionist Women's Organization "Hadassah" (established on Purim in 1907). This signaled the inauguration of Hadassah's practical activity which set as its goal the eradication of infectious diseases, helping set up health stations, and assisting the woman of Jerusalem. At the end of World War I, Hadassah sent a medical delegation to help establish medical institutions in the land of Israel. That same year, 1918, Hadassah established a nursing school in Jerusalem. The university hospital on Mount Scopus was founded only in 1939 and was in fact the first medical school in the land of Israel.

Other institutions of healing

Other ethnic communities also maintained institutions of healing in Jerusalem. Especially noteworthy is the research work of Norbert Schwake on the development of hospitals in Jerusalem from the eighteenth century to the beginning of the twentieth, as well as the descriptions of Swiss physician Titus Tobler. He refers to several Muslim and smaller hospitals in the middle of the nineteenth century (such as the hospital for the poor in the Tekiyeh building), that could not be included in the category of modern hospitals. In addition, the Catholics (Franciscans) had the Dar Ishaq Bek that served as a shelter for the poor and sick alike. Likewise Jerusalem had within its city limits hospitals for Christians of all nationalities, such as: the English Missionary Hospital which began operations in 1844, the Prussian Hospital at the Deaconesses' House, and the French Hospital which was founded in 1851.

The development of the new city of Jerusalem outside the city walls brought about a momentum of construction, and people of different nationalities also wished to leave heir mark and impact on this process. Towards the end of the nineteenth century many hospitals were built, while some of them moved from the old city to the new part of the city. Of the hospitals that were built we will mention: The Children's Hospital of Dr. Carl Sadreczki (1872), the Italian Hospital (1900), and the Russian Hospital. The Lepers Hospital, which had been supported by the imperial administration, was established in 1875 near Bir Ayub and another leperosorium was built on Mamilla Street in 1866 and was administered by Dr. Tappe. This institution had already moved to its new location by 1888, to a building erected by a German Protestant Association. The German hospital (the Ziv Hospital) on the corner of Nevi'im and Strauss Streets was inaugurated in 1894 after moving outside of the city walls. Similarly the French hospital known as "Saint Louis" (on Shivtei Israel Street) which was inaugurated in 1881 (the construction was completed in 1896) was moved from the Jewish Quarter at the end of the nineteenth century. Also worthy of mention is the English St. John's Ophthalmologic Hospital (in the Valley of Ben Hinnom) which was built in 1882 and due to its importance was also recognized by the Turkish emperor.

Selected bibliography for this chapter

Ben-Arieh; Eliav, pp. 232-282, 421-423; Freidin; Gat; Haggai; Kass; Leibowitz; Levi, History; Margalit, Way, pp. 286-288; Morgenstern; Nahamias; Neumann, Medicine; Schur, History, pp. 693-695; Schwake, Development; Schwake, Hospitals; Shvartz; Stern; Tobler, Medicine; Vilnay, pp. 173-186.

PART TWO

Physicians in Jerusalem in the Tenth to Eighteenth Centuries

This section includes a list of physicians (accompanied by a brief accompanying bibliography) who were active in Jerusalem in the tenth-eighteenth centuries. The list is based on a variety of written sources dealing with the history of physicians and medicine in general, historical chronicles, travel journals, and diverse documents. From the Ottoman Period onward, the Ottoman and Franciscan archives, the Responsa literature, and the records of the Muslim courts in Jerusalem must be cited for their contribution.

The list is incomplete and the quality of information on a number of physicians, their status, and activity is limited, depending on the historical information available to the author. Thus, missing from the list are the names of physicians from Jerusalem in the earlier centuries, despite the fact that unquestionably there were physicians at work during those periods. This reflects the paucity of historical information on the land of Israel and Jerusalem in particular in those centuries. On the other hand, the relatively long list of physicians mentioned in Jerusalem in the sixteenth – eighteenth centuries is, to a large extent, the product of a wealth of available extant sources from that period. The quantity of sources is also connected with the relative importance of Jerusalem in various periods. Thus, for example, the scarcity of sources on physicians in Jerusalem during the Mamluk Period reflects its inferior status in the eyes of the Mamluk ruling authority.

The list includes only those physicians who were explicitly mentioned by name in connection with Jerusalem. Although this is a partial list, one may learn much from it about the origins of the physicians, as well as their professional training, and generally more about the nature of medicine in Jerusalem. These subjects were treated in the first section of the book. Not included in the list are the names of the Franciscan physicians who lived in Jerusalem in the sixteenth-eighteenth centuries, and they appear in a separate table in the chapter on medicine in Jerusalem in the Ottoman Period (Section I, chapter seven).

1. Yusuf al-Nasrani

Yusuf al-Nasrani was a famous Christian physician who was also an expert in other fields of science. Ca. 980 Caliph Fatimid al-'Aziz appointed Yusuf al-Nasrani to the position of patriarch in Jerusalem. He served in this position for three years and eight months. He died in Egypt.[1]

2. al-Hassan ibn Muhamd abi Na'im

Al-Hassan ibn Muhamd abi Na'im 'Ali al-Tabib, a Jerusalem physician of the tenth century.[2]

[1] Ibn abi Usaybi'a, p. 545.
[2] Ibn al-Qifti, p. 169.

3. Anaba Zekhryah ibn Thuaba

A tenth-century Christian monk of Jerusalem, he possessed extensive knowledge in the sciences and in medicine and served as teacher to the noted Jerusalem physician, al-Tamimi.[3]

4. al-Tamimi

Abu 'Abdalla Muhamd ibn Sa'ed al-Tamimi, a Muslim, who lived in the second half of the tenth century. Al-Tamimi was a native of Jerusalem where he also acquired his medical training. After completing his apprenticeship in Ramle, he moved to Egypt ca. 980, where he was close to the vizier Ya'qub ibn Killis (930-991) who worked on behalf of Caliph Fatimid al-M'uz and his son al-'Aziz. Al-Tamimi wrote many medical works, the large part of which are no longer in existence today. Part of his well-known treatise, known in brief as "al-Murshed" (the guide), has remained in manuscript form, as yet unpublished, and other parts are quoted by later writers such as Maimonides and Ibn al-Baytar. Al-Tamimi specialized particularly in the subject of "theriac" and ophthalmology and is the most important source for learning about the various materia medica that were in use in al-Sham during the First Muslim Period (until 1099). He refers among others to medicinal herbs used by the residents of Jerusalem and the environs for eating and medical purposes, among them: Silybum marianum, Sisymbrium officinale, and Coronopus squamatus. In his treatise there are many references to realia, the daily life of the local residents and their beliefs, especially in the greater Jerusalem area and the Dead Sea basin. [4]

5. Slama Ibn al-Muqaddasi (of Jerusalem) al-Theriaqi

Physician and Muslim cleric who was active in Jerusalem in the tenth century. His sobriquet "al-Theriaqi" attests to his expertise in preparing the theriac compound.[5]

6. Roberto the Physician

Known in Latin as Roberto medico, a twelfth-century Frankish physician, who lived for many years with his family in Jerusalem near the Pool of the Patriarch. He may have been a native of the land of Israel.[6]

7. William the Physician

Known in Latin as Willelmo medico, mentioned in a document from 1138 as a property-owner in Jerusalem.[7]

8. Benevenutus Grapheus of Jerusalem

Lived during the Crusader Period in the Kingdom of Jerusalem (12th-13th centuries). He is not mentioned in the historical literature despite the fact that he wrote an important treatise on ophthalmology which

---

[3] Ibn abi Usaybi'a, p. 546.

[4] Ibn abi Usaybi'a, pp. 546-548; Ibn al-Qifti. pp. 105-106; Leclerc, I, pp. 388-391; Amar, Tradition, pp. 23-34.

[5] Ibn al-Atir, al-Lubab, p. 214.

[6] Röhricht, Regesta, doc. no. 170, p. 42 (dated 1137); nos. 430-431, p. 112 (dated 1167); Wickersheimer, p. 692.

[7] Röhricht, Regesta, doc. no. 182, p. 45.

influenced medical culture in Europe. It is not even known whether he was a Jew or a Christian. In his book he calls himself "of Jerusalem" and makes many references to "our Jerusalem medicines".[8]

9. Abu Suliman Daud

Abu Suliman Daud ibn al-Mani ibn Abi Fana, a Muslim physician and astrologist who converted to Christianity; he apparently came from Egypt. In one of the first invasions by the Crusader King Amalrich I (ruled 1162-1174), the king met the physician and was impressed by his medical talents. Amalrich sent him with his five children to Jerusalem. Abu Suliman attended Amalrich's son, Baldwin IV, who was afflicted with leprosy. The son of Abu Suliman, Abu al-Khair, grew up and was educated in Jerusalem together with Baldwin IV and became a Crusader knight, while the other four sons practiced medicine in the service of various Ayyubid rulers. It is reported that Abu Suliman told the Ayyubid ruler Saladin in 1184 that according to his astrological predictions, he would conquer Jerusalem. When Saladin ultimately did conquer Jerusalem from the Franks in 1187, he remembered the physician favorably and treated him and his family who were living in Jerusalem with great kindness. A short time afterwards, Abu Suliman died.[9]

10. Abu Sa'ed

Abu Sa'ed was the eldest son of Abu Suliman who served as court physician to the Frankish king, Amalrich I.[10]

11. Eliyahu ben Zekhariya

Eliyahu ben Zekhariya (known as Abu al-Faraj of Alexandria) was a judge and physician, whose family came from Egypt. He lived between 1160-1242 approximately. Eliyahu ben Zekhariya was active in the land of Israel and lived for many years in Jerusalem with his wife and children, close upon Saladin's conquest of the city. He may have served as a physician for Malik al-Kamil. His two sons also practiced medicine: Abu Zekri, an eye doctor, worked in Egypt as well as Jerusalem, and another son was either a physician or a physician's assistant in the city of Acre.[11]

12. Abu Zekri

Abu Zekri ben Eliyahu was the personal physician to Sultan al-Malik al-'Aziz. He was the son of Eliyahu ben Zekhariya, the physician who lived in Jerusalem for many years, and he, too, lived there in 1196, as part of his work for sultans al-Malik al-'Aziz and al-Malik al-Mu'azzam 'Isa. Abu Zekri served principally as an eye doctor.[12]

---

[8] Kedar, Benevenutus, pp. 14-41.
[9] Ibn abi Usaybi'a, pp. 587-589; Cahen, pp. 351-360.
[10] Ibn abi Usaybi'a, p. 588.
[11] Goitein, Jewry, pp. 261-263, 322, fn. 8; Motzkin, p. 344.
[12] Goitein, Jewry, pp. 262-275, 321-326; Motzkin, p. 344-349.

13. Abu Mansur

Sheikh Abu Mansur was a Christian physician who lived in Jerusalem in the Ayyubid Period.[13]

14. Muwaffaq al-Din Ya'qub ibn Siqlab

Muwaffaq al-Din Ya'qub ibn Siqlab, a Christian, was a native of Jerusalem, who lived there for many years. He acquired his medical training in Jerusalem and the environs from other physicians. He was considered in his time an expert on the writings of Galenius and served as a practicing physician at the hospital in Jerusalem and as a consultant to the Ayyubid ruler al-Mu'azzam 'Isa. (ruled 1218-1228). A short time after the sultan's death, Ya'qub ibn Siqlab died in Damascus, in 1228.[14]

15. Rashid al-Din Abu Sa'ed

Rashid al-Din Abu Sa'ed, a Christian expert physician, also renowned for his knowledge of the Arabic language. He was the son of the physician Muwaffaq al-Din Ya'qub and like his father, was a resident of Jerusalem and served the various Ayyubid rulers: al-Mu'azzam 'Isa (ruled 1218-1228), from 1234 onward, he attended al-Kamil, and then served for nine years as physician to al-Salih Najm al-Din Ayyub (1240-1249). He even wrote one of his medical treatises for al-Salih Najm al-Din.[15]

16. Sadid al-Din Abu Mansur

Sadid al-Din Abu Mansur was a Christian physician who converted to Islam and became an important expert on Muslim law. He was also a son of the physician, Muwaffaq al-Din Ya'qub. He served in the city of Karak under the Ayyubid ruler al-Nasir Daud, and died in Damascus.[16]

17. 'Abd al-Latif al-Baghdadi

Muwaffaq al-Din 'Abd al-Latif al-Baghdadi (1162-1231) was a Moslem physician who came from Baghdad. He was expert in various sciences and also achieved renown as a religious scholar. In Damascus he taught medicine. In 1191 he met with Saladin in Jerusalem and witnessed the entrenchment activities against the crusader onslaughts. He also lived in Egypt for several years where he met Maimonides. Abd al-Latif returned to Jerusalem ca. 1202 where he taught the various sciences and visited the al-Aqsa mosque frequently. Abd al-Latif al-Baghdadi wrote many books, including one written in the city of Jerusalem in 1207.[17]

---

[13] Ibn abi Usaybi'a, p. 698.
[14] Ibn abi Usaybi'a, p. 697-699; Ibn al-Qifti, pp. 378-379; Kohlberg & Kedar, pp. 113-126.
[15] Ibn abi Usaybi'a, pp. 599-600.
[16] Ibn abi Usaybi'a, p. 699.
[17] Ibn abi Usaybi'a, pp. 683-694; Bagdadi, pp. 5-7; Klein-Franke, p. 127.

18. Rashid al-Din al-Suri

Rashid al-Din ibn al-Suri (1178-1242) was a physician from Tyre, who was considered a great expert in knowledge of the different drugs, their names and properties, and he wrote books on the subject. He lived in Jerusalem for two years and served as a physician at the hospital there. The Ayyubid ruler al-'Adil (1218) brought him to Egypt from Jerusalem in 1216 to act as his personal physician. After the death of al-'Adil, he served al-Mu'azzam 'Isa (ruled 1218-1228) and al-Nasir Daud. Later Rashid al-Din al-Suri moved to Damascus, where he established a council of sages on the subject of medicine and he died in the city in 1242.[18]

19. Abu al-'Abbas al-Giyani

Sheikh Abu al-'Abbas al-Giyani, a Muslim physician, who specialized in "unique drugs" and additional fields of science, is mentioned as one of the physicians under whom the physician Ibn al-Suri trained during his stay in Jerusalem, apparently between 1214-1216.[19]

20. Abu al-'Abbas al-Nabati

Abu al-'Abbas was an Andalusian Muslim physician and herbalist. He was born in Seville ca. 1165 and according to another opinion, in 1172. In his native country, he was renowned as a distinguished scholar of religious law, but above all, became famous for his outstanding knowledge of medicinal herbs and their uses, thus his sobriquet: "al-Nabati" (the herbalist). In early 1215 Abu al-'Abbas began his long journey to the Orient, which took several years, during which he also came to al-Sham. Abu al-'Abbas described many plants from the land of Israel, and he mentioned the Jerusalem region many times. This would indicate that he stayed in the area for a relatively extended period, which enabled him to become very familiar with the flora of the city. Among the plants from the Jerusalem region mentioned are: Reseda alba, Asphodelus ramosus, and Sarcopoterium spinosa. Abu al-'Abbas returned to Spain from this expedition in 1228 and died there in 1239. His treatise has not survived but excerpts from it are quoted in a book written by his distinguished pupil, Ibn al-Baytar.[20]

21. Ibn al-Baytar

Abu Muhamd Abd Allah Ibn Ahmed Ibn al-Baytar was born ca. 1197 in the city of Malaga, in southern Spain. In his youth he studied botany and medicine under Abu al-'Abbas al-Nabati. In 1219 at the age of twenty, Ibn al-Baytar went on an extended study expedition to various countries around the Mediterranean basin where he studied the science of medicine and botany with the foremost physicians and herbalists. At the end of his expedition he arrived in Egypt and served in the court of the Ayyubid ruler al-Kamil ibn al-'Adil as chief physician to the sultan. In 1240, some two years after the death of al-Kamil, Ibn al-Baytar

[18] Ibn abi Usaybi'a, pp. 699-703.
[19] Ibn abi Usaybi'a, p. 700.
[20] al-Maqqari, II, p. 596; Leclerc, II, pp. 244-248; Amar, Herbalist, pp. 235-239.

continued his position in Damascus for the last Ayyubid ruler, al-Salih Najm al-Din Ayyub. As part of his duties for the Ayyubid rulers, Ibn al-Baytar pursued a more extensive study of the plants in al-Sham. The descriptions and variety of scenes mentioned in his books demonstrate that he had a first-hand knowledge of the nature and flora of the country which he acquired during his travels through the countryside for research purposes.

The most famous of his works is "The Collection of Simple Drugs" which contains a vast quantity of material, almost all of the applied knowledge in botanical medicine up until his times. In this treatise Ibn al-Baytar refers to the many medicinal plants from the Jerusalem area with which he must have been personally familiar. He also quotes excerpts from other physicians and other earlier, forgotten medical treatises in his work, which contain extensive material about the medical substances in Jerusalem.[21]

22. Nachmanides

R. Moshe ben Nachman, or Nachmanides (1194-1270) was born in Gerona, Spain, one of the greatest Jewish scholars of the Middle Ages. He was known primarily for his important commentary on the Pentateuch, embedded with a vast treasury of information about his medical and scientific knowledge. Although we do not possess any specific medical treatises written by him, some scholars believe that he was a physician or healer and even practiced medicine. He immigrated to the land of Israel in 1267 and contributed greatly to the establishment of the Jewish community in Jerusalem. It is noteworthy that Nachmanides' personal seal was found close to Tel Kisan in the Valley of Acre and there are accounts that when he lived in Spain, he used the seals for medicinal purposes.[22]

23. Nagm al-Din ibn al-Labudi

Nagm al-Din ibn al-Labudi, Muslim physician, scion of a family of physicians, was born in Aleppo in 1211 and grew up in Damascus. He was considered an expert physician and also was proficient in other fields of science. He served as physician to various Ayyubid rulers and also took part in important administrative functions: he was appointed vizier and officer in charge of the taxation office in Egypt, and later in greater Syria. It is known that he lived in Jerusalem in 1268.[23]

24. 'Ismael ibn Ibrahim ibn Suliman al-Muqaddasi

'Ismael ibn Ibrahim ibn Suliman al-Muqaddasi, a physician who came from Jerusalem, as his name attests, was the pupil of Muhamd 'Imad al-Din al-Nablussi (who in his last years served as qadi of Jerusalem, where he died in 1336) and later moved to Jerusalem. It was said of him that he showed great interest in medicine

[21] Ibn abi Usaybi'a, pp. 601-602; al-Maqqari, II, pp. 691-692; Amar, Ibn al-Baytar, pp. 49-76.
[22] Margalit, Ramban, pp. 303-315; Shachar, Seal, pp. 146-147.
[23] Ibn abi Usaybi'a, p. 666.

and even practiced it, and was considered a superb healer. He died in 1331.[24]

25. Me'ir Aldabi

R. Me'ir ibn Aldabi, Jewish physician and philosopher, was the grandson of a renowned Talmud commentator the "Rosh" (Rabbeinu Asher), born in Toledo, probably in 1310. In his book 'Shevile Emunah' (The Paths of Faith) written ca. 1360, he devotes sizable sections to medical subjects. At the end of his treatise, R. Me'ir Aldabi writes that it was written in Jerusalem. We have no other source to confirm this information.[25]

26. Avraham Halevi

Avraham Halevi, a fourteenth-century Karaite physician. His son Shmuel was named 'al-Qudsi' attesting to his Jerusalem origins.[26]

27. Baptista de Lubeck

Physician of German origin, who bore the title "Hospital Commissioner", on behalf of the Franciscan Custodian on Mt. Zion ca. 1480. He gave medical care to crusaders who fell ill when visiting Jerusalem. Thus, for example, Felix Fabri reported that Baptista tended him when he suffered from pains and a high fever, due to overeating melons on his visit to Jerusalem.[27]

28. R. Moshe Vidalish

R. Moshe Vidalish the physician immigrated to Jerusalem apparently at the beginning of the sixteenth century. He was a well-to-do individual who purchased many properties in Jerusalem. He is referred to by the title "the physician" in the will that he drew up in 1502.[28]

29. Yitzhak Harofe

The surgeon Yitzhak, a native of Jerusalem was a physician in Krakow in 1507.[29]

30. R. David ibn Shushan

R. David ibn Shushan was the head of the Sephardic yeshiva in Jerusalem at the beginning of the sixteenth century. He also served as physician to the Jewish community. R. Yisrael Ashkenazi mentions him in a letter he wrote from Jerusalem in 1522: "But he also practices medicine".[30]

---

[24] al-'Asqalani, I, p. 387.
[25] Zonta, pp. 278-279.
[26] Mann, II, p. 142; Strauss, p. 556.
[27] Arce, p. 123; Felix Fabri, in: PPTS 9-10, p. 113.
[28] Responsa Ralbah, par. 25.
[29] Gelber, p. 348.
[30] Basola, p. 62; David, Letter, p. 121; David, Immigration, p. 166.

31. R. Shlomo Lurie

R. Shlomo Lurie of Lublin was a physician as well as an outstanding Torah scholar and kabbalist. He immigrated to Israel ca. 1570 at the age of 80 and settled in Jerusalem.[31]

32. R. Shmuel Halevi

R. Shmuel Halevi the elder was apparently R. Shmuel ben Hakim (=the physician). He practiced medicine in Egypt and using the proceeds of his labors, purchased property in Jerusalem. R. Shmuel Halevi immigrated to the land of Israel and was one of the rabbis of Jerusalem in the first half of the sixteenth century.[32]

33. 'Abd al-Karim ibn Musa

'Abd al-Karim ibn Musa, a Jewish-Karaite physician, who practiced medicine in Jerusalem between 1532-1552. He was a leader of the Jewish Karaite community and served as commissioner of the charitable trust for the Jewish community in Jerusalem. He achieved the senior professional position of "head of the physicians" in Jerusalem. He substituted for the head of the physicians at the Jerusalem Hospital when the latter was forced to travel to Istanbul in 1547 for several months.[33]

34. Ibrahim ben Shumali

A Jewish physician who was active in Jerusalem, mentioned in a document from 1542 in relation to treatment he gave a Muslim patient.[34]

35. Yehudah ben Musa

Yehudah ben Musa (=Moses) ben Ya'akov, a Jewish physician, is mentioned in a document from 1548, in the context of the sale of an orchard in Malha (a village near Jerusalem) to a Muslim.[35]

36. Yosef ben Ibrahim

A Jewish physician who practiced medicine in Jerusalem between 1552-1578. His family origins were in Alexandria. The sources show that this physician and his family owned much property in Jerusalem.[36]

37. 'Abd al-Karim ibn 'Abd al-Latif

'Abd al-Karim ibn 'Abd al-Latif, a Jewish-Karaite physician who practiced medicine in Jerusalem between 1550-1561.[37]

---

[31] Frumkin-Rivlin, I, p. 115.
[32] Radbaz, par. A(272); Responsa Ralbah, par. 61; Frumkin-Rivlin, I, p. 89.
[33] Cohen, Jewish, pp. 188-191; Cohen, 16th Century, p. 284, no. 322; p. 298, no. 339; p. 327. no. 371.
[34] Cohen, Jewish, p. 189.
[35] Cohen, 16th Century, pp. 308-309, no. 351.
[36] Cohen, Jewish, pp. 188-191.
[37] Cohen, Jewish, pp. 188-189; 16th Century, p. 99, no. 92.

38. Ya'aqub the Physician

A Jewish physician by the name of Ya'aqub is mentioned in a document of the Muslim court from 8.1.1550. He rented a shop in Jerusalem from the Muslim waqf which he used as a clinic.[38]

39. Musa the Physician

Musa (=Moses) the physician of Jerusalem served as authorized agent for Ya'aqub the physician. He is mentioned in a document from 8.1.1550.[39]

40. Shmuel the Physician

Shmuel the physician from Jerusalem served as authorized agent for Ya'aqub the physician together with Musa the physician. He is mentioned in a document from 8.1.1550.[40]

41. Barbosa the Physician

A famous physician, born in Portugal who left Christianity and converted to Judaism. He sailed to Ancona and from there to Turkey, eventually settling down in the Jewish community in Jerusalem. The Portuguese traveler Panteleo di Avero met him in Jerusalem ca. 1560 and noted: "...Barbosa, and he is an eminent physician". Amatus Luzitanus described him in an essay on medicine as "an excellent, learned physician with long experience".[41]

42. Suliman ben Ya'aqub

A Jewish physician from Jerusalem, mentioned in a document from 1563 related to leasing his shop, which was located near the 'Chain Gate', to a Muslim.[42]

43. Yehie the Physician

Yehie son of Yosef son of Salmon, a Jewish physician, certified by the court of the Ottoman Sultan in Istanbul. He specialized in medicine and intuitive physiognomy. Yehie received approval for his application of 29.10.1564 to practice medicine in Jerusalem and even received a regular salary from the state treasury.[43]

44. Suliman ben 'Ali

Suliman was the son of 'Ali the physician, who lived in the Jewish neighborhood. Because of improper

[38] Cohen, 16th Century, p. 269, no. 302.
[39] Cohen, 16th Century, p. 269, no. 302.
[40] Cohen, 16th Century, p. 269, no. 302.
[41] Slushatz, Community, p. 328; Rozen, Community, p. 232; Schur, Community, p. 362, fn. 27.
[42] Cohen, Jewish, p. 211,n. 189. This apparently is Salmon al-Tabib mentioned in another document of the Moslem religious courts from that year together with David ben Zamir Hadayan , (apparently the Radvaz!) , see: Joshua, p. 276. He may have been the son of Ya'aqub the physician, see: Cohen, 16th Century, p. 269, no. 302.
[43] Cohen, 16th Century, pp. 269-270, no. 303; Cohen, Jewish, p. 190.

behavior, the qadi of Jerusalem ordered him to leave the neighborhood on 4.12.1564.[44]

45. Kamal ibn Musa

Kamal ibn Musa was a Jewish eye doctor who worked in Jerusalem and even served as a rabbinical judge in the Jewish community. His clinic was located in the 'Attarin market in a shop that he leased for a year (where he was preceded by a Muslim physician). As a medical specialist and "head of the physicians" in Jerusalem, he received a salary from the public coffers and when he asked to leave Jerusalem for a short period, was compelled to receive permission from his superiors and to find a suitable replacement. The approval was granted on 16.7.1571.[45]

46. 'Imad al-Din ibn Shams al-Din Muhamd ibn Muslem

Sheikh 'Imad al-Din ibn Shams al-Din Muhamd ibn Muslem was an eye doctor in Jerusalem. On 16.7.1571 he received a temporary appointment as a public doctor receiving a salary. 'Imad al-Din the physician is also mentioned in a document from 1578.[46]

47. Yosef ben Ishaq

Yosef ben Ishaq (=Yitzhak), a Jewish physician, with a high professional ranking, who worked in Jerusalem. He is mentioned in a document from 1575.[47]

48. Shhada ben Ibrahim

Shhada ben Ibrahim, a Jewish physician, practiced medicine in Jerusalem even though he had not completed his medical training. He was warned by the Muslim qadi on 25.3.1577 not to practice ophthalmology or eye surgery until he studied surgery. In a later date, from 1581-1583 he is referred to as "the eye doctor" and it seems that by this time, he had already received his official certification. Shhada ben Ibrahim lived in the Jewish neighborhood in Jerusalem.[48]

49. Muhamd ibn Ahmad

Muhamd ibn Ahmad was the head of the surgeons in Jerusalem, and his father held this office before him. As part of his duties, he was responsible for maintaining the professional standards of the physicians who performed surgery in the city of Jerusalem.[49]

[44] Cohen, 16th Century, p. 270, no. 304; Cohen, Jewish, p. 192.
[45] Cohen, 16th Century, p. 12, no. 7, p. 271, no. 305; Cohen, Jewish, p. 50-51, 190-191.
[46] Cohen, 16th Century, p. 271, no. 305; Richard, Jerusalem, p. 78.
[47] Cohen, Jewish, p. 191.
[48] Cohen, 16th Century, p. 59, no. 57, p. 166, no. 171; p. 271, no. 306; Cohen, Jewish, p. 189.
[49] Cohen, 16th Century, p. 271, no. 306, (dated 25.3.1577).

50. R' Hayyim Vital

R. Hayyim ben Yosef Vital (1543-1620) was apparently born in Safad and his family origins were probably in Italy. One of the scholars and kabbalists of Safad in the second half of the sixteenth century, he was considered the outstanding and most important pupil of the "Ari". R. Hayyim Vital moved to Jerusalem for several years, living there alternately between 1577-1584 and 1591-1594 approximately and engaged in Torah scholarship and kabbalah. Beyond this, he was apparently also engaged in other sciences: alchemy, astronomy, and medicine, even writing a book of remedies when he lived in Damascus (ca. 1610-1620). This was after the period that he lived in Jerusalem where he apparently did not practice medicine at all.[50]

51. Daud al-Antaki

Daud ibn Amar al-Antaki was a Muslim physician, blind from birth. He was born in Antioch where he studied mathematics and natural sciences. After the death of his father, he studied medicine in Cairo and primarily in Damascus. His books refer to the many materia medica that came from Jerusalem and it seems that some of the knowledge that he brings was acquired personally. His treatise reflects the earliest introduction of European culture and its effect on the Orient on the one hand, and represents the swan song of the celebrated Muslim medical culture on the other. He died in 1599.[51]

52. R. Yitzhak the Physician

R. Yitzhak the physician was one of the two regular physicians of Jerusalem at the beginning of the seventeenth century and is mentioned in Franciscan chronicles of January 1612. It may be that this person is R. Yitzhak Ispania (the Spaniard) a distinguished physician who came to Jerusalem from Constantinople and settled there at that time.[52]

53. Cacya 'Ali

In the Franciscan chronicles a physician and scholar is mentioned in January of 1612 by the name of Cacya Haly as one of the two regular physicians of Jerusalem at that time.[53]

54. Johann of Bergamo

A Christian physician from the Franciscans who served in Jerusalem. In 1612 he was called to attend the mufti of Jerusalem, during the absence of the city's regular physicians.[54]

---

[50] Benayahu, Jerusalem, pp. 65-75; David, Immigration, p. 167; Behayahu, Anthology, pp. 91-112; Benayahu, Medicine, pp. 3-17.
[51] al-Antaki; al-Muhibbi, II, pp. 141-142;. Plessner, pp. 138-141.
[52] Boucher, p. 295; Conforote, p. 49; Frumkin-Rivlin, I, p. 35; Koren, p. 64.
[53] Boucher, p. 295.
[54] Boucher, p. 296.

55. R. Ya'akov ibn 'Amram

R. Ya'akov ibn 'Amram, one of the heads and leaders of the Jewish community in Jerusalem in the first half of the seventeenth century, who apparently died there before 1650. He is called "the physician" and in one of the sources "Doctor Ya'akov ben 'Amram".[55]

56. R. Ya'akov Abuhav

R. Ya'akov Abuhav the physician was one of Jerusalem's scholars during the rule of Muhamd ibn Farukh (1625-1627).[56]

57. R. Raphael Abuhav

R. Raphael Abuhav, physician and rabbinical court judge in the Jewish community of Jerusalem in the first half of the seventeenth century.[57]

58. Yitzhak Havilio

Yitzhak Havilio the physician, one of the heads of the Jewish community in Jerusalem during the reign of the despot Muhamd ibn Farukh (1625-1627).[58]

59. Shmuel Halevi

Shmuel Halevi, physician to Uthaman Aga (brother-in-law of ibn Farukh) and of the governor of Gaza. Acted as intercessor on behalf of the Jewish community during the despotic rule of Muhamd ibn Farukh (1625-1627) and was even imprisoned in Jerusalem for his efforts.[59]

60. R. Ya'akov Tzemakh

R. Ya'akov Tzemakh, a Marrano from Portugal who returned to Judaism in Saloniki at the age of 35. He immigrated to the land of Israel ca. 1619, settling in Jerusalem and engaging in the study of kabbalah. R. Ya'akov acquired a reputation as a "distinguished physician" and even served as personal physician to the governor of Safad.[60]

61. Yehudah Mr'ali

Yehudah Mr'ali, a Jerusalem physician of North-African origin, was the pupil of R. Yitzhak Sabach, one of the scholars of Jerusalem in the first half of the seventeenth century.[61]

---

[55] Rozen, Ruins, p. 91, fn. 60, pp. 113, 126-127, 130-131.
[56] Rozen, Ruins, p. 110.
[57] Rozen, Ruins, p. 110. fn. 268.
[58] Rozen, Ruins, p. 104. fn. 190.
[59] Rozen, Ruins, p. 117.
[60] Conforote, p. 49; Shalom, pp. 185-194.
[61] Rozen, Community, p. 96.

62. R. Avraham Hacohen

R. Avraham Hacohen the physician was born ca. 1543 in the city of Fez in North Africa. He was considered one of Morocco's most eminent rabbis. He immigrated to Jerusalem in 1653 at the age of 110 and taught Torah there. After three-four months, he died in Jerusalem.[62]

63. Mozes Mechaelius

Mozes Mechaelius of Jerusalem is mentioned in the records of Leiden University in 1658.[63]

64. R. Ya'akov Hajiz

R. Ya'akov Hajiz (1620-1674) one of the great scholars of Jerusalem in the seventeenth century. He was born in Fez and in his youth moved to Italy. In 1658, he immigrated to Jerusalem where he established a large center for Torah study. He also had a medical education, although it seems that he never actually practiced.[64]

65. R. Menahem Amargi

R. Menahem Amargi one of Jerusalem's scholars who was considered a "distinguished physician". He died in Jerusalem around 1670-1675.[65]

66. Maslh Galbi

Haj Maslh Galbi is mentioned as the head of the physicians in Jerusalem, in a document from 1694. By virtue of this position, he appointed the person who was in charge of the waqf of al-Bimaristan al-Salahi .[66]

67. R. Yekutiel the Physician

R. Yekiutiel son of the hassid R. Leib of Vilna had medical training. He was active in Padua, too, and was considered one of the scholars of Jerusalem at the end of the seventeenth century.[67]

68. R. Simha Menahem of Yona

R. Simha Menahem son of R. Yohanan Baruch (the physician) of Yona was a distinguished physician, scion of a family expelled from Portugal. He served as coordinator of contributions in Lvov on behalf of the Jewish community of Jerusalem.[68]

---

[62] Toledeno, p. 141; Frumkin, Rivlin, II, pp. 34-35.
[63] Kaplan, p. 66.
[64] Frumkin-Rivlin,II, p. 62, fn. 2; Ben-Zvi, pp. 250-254.
[65] Shalom, p. 188.
[66] al-'Asali, Wata'iq, pp. 90-91.
[67] Frumkin-Rivlin, II, p. 139.
[68] Ya'ari, Emissaries, p. 67; Sohastov, III, p. 27 and in all entries describing the Yona family.

69. R. Refael Mordekhai Malki

R. Refael Mordekhai Malki was born in the Iberian peninsula and lived part of his life as a Christian in Christian society; he later returned to Judaism. A large part of his life was spent in Italy and it is almost certain that he acquired his medical education and experience there. He immigrated to Jerusalem in 1677 and settled there until the end of his life in 1702. R. Refael Mordekhai Malki distinguished himself in Jerusalem as an expert on Jewish law and as a distinguished physician. He was a man of property and was one of the leaders of the Jewish community in Jerusalem. In the commentary that he wrote on the Torah, we learn much about the status of medicine in Jerusalem; about the diseases and medications that were widespread and the poor level of the physicians. He would cure patients at no charge and supported public administration of the public institution – the Bikkur Holim health fund of the Jews of Jerusalem. R. Refael Malki was summoned to treat R. Yehudah Hahasid when he fell ill upon his arrival in Jerusalem, on the first day of Heshvan in 1700. [69]

70. R. David de Silva

R. David de Silva was born and died in Jerusalem (1684-1740). He was the son of R. Hisqiya de Silva who wrote the book "P'ri Hadash" and the grandson of R. Refael Mordekhai Malki. During his first trip to Europe, (1706) he studied medicine in Holland and was certified as a distinguished physician. When he returned to Jerusalem, he practiced medicine as a livelihood and treated a variety of diseases. He was strongly influenced by Tobias Cohen the physician whom he consulted on medical matters. He wrote a treatise entitled "P'ri Hadas" (Myrtle Fruit. that deals with many subjects, primarily medicine. This treatise is presently still in manuscript form, and this author is working diligently to publish it.[70]

71. R. Mordekhai the Physician

R. Mordekhai the physician a leader of the Sephardic Jewish community in Jerusalem is mentioned in records of the Muslim court in the first third of the eighteenth century. Mordekhai was a surgeon and one of his treatments caused damage to a Muslim patient; in consequence he was compelled to pay a monetary compensation.[71]

72. Salmon the Physician

R. Salmon was one of the leaders of the Sephardic Jewish community in Jerusalem at the beginning of the eighteenth century. He is referred to as a physician in a document from 1711, in relation to a treatment for a sick pregnant woman from the village of Silwan. Her husband accused him before the Muslim court of having given the woman to drink leaves of Cassia acutifolia (alexandria), which caused her to miscarry and

[69] Malki, pp. 11-19, 44-48; Rozen, Community, pp. 170-171; Rozen, Identity, pp. 19-23; Rozen and Vitztum, pp. 75-77; Singer, p. 200; Ya'ari, Travels, p. 328.
[70] Pri Hadas; Frumkin-Rivlin, II, pp. 106-107; David, Collection, p. 109.
[71] Cohen, 18th Century, no. 238, pp. 279-280 (dated 1702); no. 282, p. 327 (dated 1735).

die. For his part, Salmon the physician contended that he had ordered that the woman be given a drink of Nuphar and Cichorium. The judge accepted the physician's version of the event and acquitted him.[72]

73. Yosef the Physician

Yosef ben Alsarar (?) the Jew is described in a document from 1719 as "poor, old, and sick, and he practices medicine without hope of material reward ...he helps people, treats the Muslims with respect and cures them for altruistic reasons". This same Yosef the physician asked the central administration to intervene on his behalf with the Jewish community to prevent them from imposing excessive taxes on him.[73]

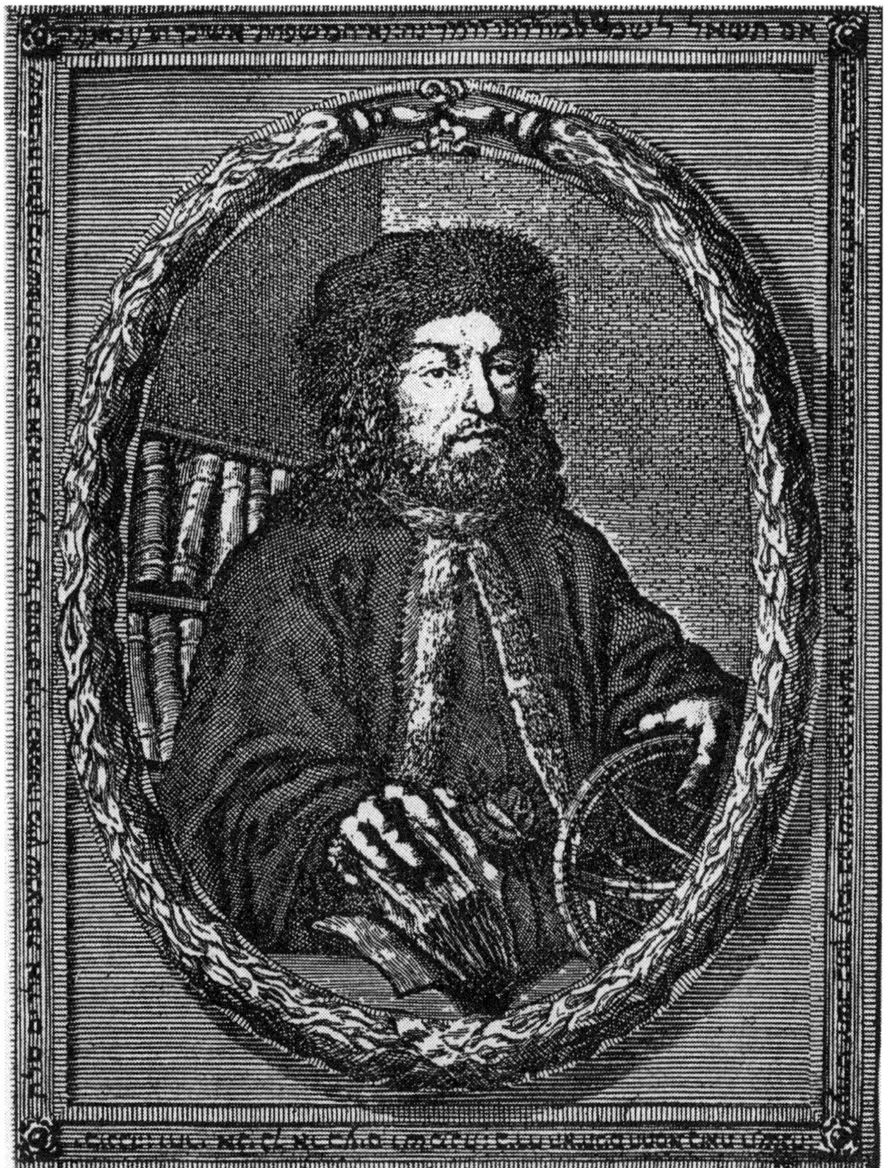

Figure 24: Portrait of R. Tobias Cohen the Physician as he appears in the frontispiece to his medical treatise "Ma'aseh Tuviyyah".

[72] Cohen, 18th Century, no. 5-6, pp. 15-16; no. 279, pp. 324-325.
[73] Cohen, 18th Century, no. 280, pp. 326.

74. Tobias Cohen the Physician

R. Tobias Cohen (Katz) the physician (1652-1729) was born in Metz. As a youth he moved to Poland. He received his medical education in Italy and returned to Poland where he practiced medicine for many years, also serving as physician to several ministers of the Ottoman Emperor. In 1701 he completed his medical treatise "Ma'aseh Tuviyyah" (published in Venice only in 1707) which is considered one of the most important scientific works written at that time. Tobias the physician immigrated to Jerusalem, probably in 1708, where his only daughter, from his second wife, was born; he later married off this daughter to R. Avraham ben Shmuel Meyuhas, one of Jerusalem's Torah scholars. After his first trip to Jerusalem, R. Tobias returned to Constantinople for several years. In 1715, at the age of 62, he returned to Jerusalem. He was involved in the civic activities of the Jewish community in the city and lived there until his death. After being stricken with paralysis, he died and was buried in the Valley of Jehosophat on 24.12.1729.[74] (Fig. 24)

75. R. Eliyau ibn Shangi

R. Eliyahu in Shangi was an prominent physician who served as medical consultant to the Ottoman sultan. In his waning years, he immigrated to the land of Israel and studied Torah in Jerusalem, where he died in 1728.[75]

76. Hayyim the Surgeon

"Hayyim the Jewish Sephardic surgeon" is mentioned in a document from 1738, when he was sued by a Christian patient for damage to his eyes, following treatment.[76]

77. Castelli the Physician

Castelli was a Muslim physician, an expert surgeon, who is mentioned in a document from 1738.[77]

78. Fadhli the Physician

Fadhli the physician was a Muslim who was appointed chief physician of Jerusalem. In a document from 1740, he is referred to as an expert physician who was part of the official investigation commission that investigated the suicide of a Jew. After examining the body, he determined the circumstances of death.[78]

79. Avraham Dayan the Physician

Avraham Dyan (Dayan), a Jewish physician of Jerusalem, died in Sidon. His wife was required to pay his debts in 1745.[79]

---

[74] Frumkin-Rivlin, II, pp. 113-119; Margalit, pp. 128-131, 382-388; P'ri Hadas, p. 107a; Horn, pp. 179-180.
[75] Frumkin-Rivlin, II, p. 158.
[76] Cohen, 18th Century, no. 283, pp. 327.
[77] Cohen, 18th Century, no. 283, pp. 327.
[78] Cohen, 18th Century, no. 270, pp. 312.
[79] Cohen, 18th Century, no. 284, pp. 328.

80. Yosef Basha the Surgeon

Haj Yosef Basha, a Muslim physician, is mentioned in a document from 1748 as an expert surgeon in Jerusalem. He was called in to examine the body of a Jew who was murdered.[80]

81. 'Abd al-ghanam

In a document from 1748 there is reference to one 'Abd al-ghanam (or 'Abd al-fatah) as the chief surgeon of the city of Jerusalem. He examined the body of a Jewish woman and determined the circumstances of her death.[81]

82. Ibrahim the Physician

Ibrahim (= Avraham) the physician is mentioned in a document from 1757, in connection with the treatment of a Christian patient. His son, Mu'alem Ishaq (=Yitzhak) is mentioned in a document from 1755 among the leaders of the Sephardic community in Jerusalem.[82]

83. Yitzhak the Physician

Mu'alem Ishaq son of Ibrahim the physician is mentioned in a document from 1755 among the leaders of the Sephardic community in Jerusalem. In another document from 1756 he is mentioned among the representatives of the community under the title of "Ishaq al-Tabib" (=the physician).[83]

84. R. Shmuel ibn Shangi

There is only one report on this personage, taken from the inscription on his gravestone on the Mt. of Olives: "Grave marking of the elderly dignitary, the renowned Torah scholar, a distinguished physician who brings merit to the community, our venerable teacher Shmuel ben Shangi deceased on the 4th of Sivan 5527 (1767).[84]

85. Kamal the Physician

Kamal is mentioned in a document of the Muslim court from 1767 as "one of the physicians living in Jerusalem". This document indicates that the relationship of Kamal and his son Amin with the rest of the Jewish community in Jerusalem was inimical. They appealed to the central imperial administration in Istanbul to prevent the Jewish community from harming them and their appeal was accepted. It seems that Kamal the physician was not a native of Jerusalem and was sent there by the local authority to serve as a physician.[85]

---

80 Cohen, 18th Century, no. 271, pp. 313.
81 Cohen, 18th Century, no. 273, p. 314.
82 Cohen, 18th Century, no. 56, p. 68; no. 285, p. 328.
83 Cohen, 18th Century, no. 56, p. 68; Yehoshua, p. 277.
84 Frumkin-Rivlin, II, p. 30. He may have been one of the sons of R. Eliyahu Ibn Shangi (no. 75).
85 Cohen, 18th Century, no. 235, pp. 274-275.

86. Yitzhak the Physician

The Torah scholar Yitzhak Piroz the physician, a Karaite, was a wealthy man from Damascus. He immigrated to Jerusalem for the third time in the mid- eighteenth century.[86]

87. Salmon the Surgeon

Salmon the Jewish surgeon is described in a document from 1784 as "an eminent expert in the art of surgery, and he possesses full knowledge of this art". This account was given by other expert surgeons when Salmon was sued for the death of a Muslim patient, who died after Salmon operated on him.[87]

88. R. Yosef Pinchas

R. Yasaf M'nahas (Yosef Pinchas), one of the rabbis of Jerusalem, is mentioned by the title of "the Jewish physician" in a document from 1785.[88]

89. R. Moshe Mordechai Meyuhas

R. Moshe Mordechai Meyuhas, Jerusalem Sephardic rabbi, served for several years as the "Rishon Lezion" (=chief Sephardic rabbi) and he never left the boundaries of the land of Israel. He was considered a skilled physician and was renowned for his medical skills among the Muslims, too. He died in 1802.[89]

---

[86] Assaf, pp. 205,216.

[87] Cohen, 18th Century, no. 287, pp. 329-330. He should not be confused with Salmon the Jewish physician who was active in Jerusalem in the beginning of the eighteenth century.

[88] Cohen, 18th Century, no. 477, p. 493,and this might be referring to R. Moshe Yosef Mordechai Meyuhas the physician, see no. 89.

[89] Frumkin-Rivlin, III, p. 183.

List of Abbreviations

A	Bibliography in Arabic
ADAJ	Annual of the Department of Antiquities of Jordan
B	Bavli (=Babylonian Talmud)
BASOR	Bulletin of the American Schools of Oriental Research.
CCLS	Corpvs Christianorvm Series Latina
EI	Encyclopaedia of Islam
H	Hebrew
IEJ	Israel Exploration Journal
LCL	The Loeb Classical Library, London - Cambridge
M	Mishnah
MIE	Memoires Presentes a L'Institut d'Egypte
PEFQS	Palestine Exploration Fund, Quarterly Statement
PG	Patrologiae Graecae
PPTS	Palestine Pilgrims Text Society, London 1887–1897
RHC	Recueil des Historiens des Croisades
Hocc	Historiens Occidentaux, Paris 1844-1895.
Hor	Historiens Orientaux, Paris 1872-1906.
T	Tosefta
Y	Yerushalmi (=Jerusalem/ Palestinian Talmud)

Bibliography

Adington, Hospital: S. Adington, "The Hospital of St. John Jerusalem", in: Z. Amar, E. Lev & J. Schwartz (eds.), *Medicine in Jerusalem Throughout the Ages*, Tel-Aviv, 1999, pp. IX–XXV.

Adington, Knowledge: S. Adgington, "Medical Knowledge in the Crusading Armies: The Evidence of Albert of Acchen and Others", In: M. Barber (ed.), *The Military Orders: Faith and Caring for the Sick*, London 1994, pp. 320–326.

Adler: M.N. Adler, *The Itinerary of Benjamin of Tudela*, London 1907.

Aharoni: Y.Aharoni, *Excavations at Ramat Rahel*, Seasons 1959-1960, Roma 1962, pp. 24-27.

al-'Asali, Ma'ahid: al-'Asali, Kamil Jamil, *Ma'ahid al-'ilm fi Bayt al-Maqdis*, 'Aman 1981.[A]

al-'Asali, Wata'iq: al-'Asali, Kamil Jamil, *Wata'iq maqdisiyya tarikhiyya*, III, 'Aman 1989. [A]

al-'Asqalani: al-'Asqalani, Ibn Hajar Ahmad ibn 'Ali, *al-Durar al-kamina fi 'a'yan al-mi'a al-tamina*, ed. M. S. 'Abd al-Haqq, Cairo 1966. [A]

al-'Umari: al-'Umari, 'Ibn Fadl Allah, *Masalik al-'absar fi mamalik al-'amsar*, ed. A. F. Sayyid, Textes Arabes et Etudes Islamiques, Tome 23, Paris 1985. [A]

al-Antaki: al-Antaki, Daud., *Tadhkirat Ula li-'Lbab wa 'l-Jami' al-Ujab al-'Aajab*, Cairo 1935. [A]

al-Bagdadi: al-Bagdadi, 'Abd al-Latif ibn Yusuf, *Kitab al-'ifada wa-al-'i'tibar*, London 1965. [A]

al-Dawadari: Ibn al-Dawadari, Abu Bakr ibn 'Abd Allah, *Kanz al-durar wa-jami' al-gurar*, Cairo 1982. [A]

al-Isfahani: al-'Isfahani, 'Imad al-Din, *al-Fath al-qussi fi l-fath al-qudsi*, ed. M. Subh, Cairo 1965. [A]

Allan: N. Allan, "Hospice to Hospital in the Near East; an Instance of Continuity and Change in Late Antiquity", *Bulletin of the History of Medicine*, 64 (1990), pp. 446–462.

al-Maqqari: al-Maqqari, 'Ahmad ibn Muhammad, *Nafh al-tib min gusn al-'Andalus al-ratib*, II, ed. I. 'Abbas, Beirut 1968.[A]

al-Muhibbi: al-Muhibbi, Muhammad 'Amin ibn Fadl Allah, *Tarikh khulasat al-'atar fi 'a'yan al-qarn al-hadi 'ašar*, II, Cairo 1867. [A]

al-Muqaddasi: al-Muqaddasi, Muhammad ibn 'Ahmad, *Kitab 'ahsan al-taqasim fi ma'rifat al-'aqalim*, ed. De Goeje, Leiden 1906. [A]

al-Qalqašandi: al-Qalqašandi, Ahmad ibn 'Ali Abu al-'Abbas, *Subh al-'a'ša fi ma'rifat al-'inša*, Cairo 1913-1919. [A]

al-Sakhawi: al-Sakhawi, Muhammad ibn 'Abd al-Rahman, *al-Daw' al-lami' li-'ahl al-qarn al-tasi'*, IV, Cairo 1934 . [A]

Amar & Lev, Survey: Z. Amar & E. Lev, *A Historical Survey of Medicinal Substances of the al-Sham Region during the Middle Ages (640-1517 CE)*, Tel-Aviv 1999.

Amar & Lev, Tobler: Z. Amar & E. Lev, "The traditional materia medica in Jerusalem according to Titus Tobler", *Harefuah*, 138 (2000), pp. 604-607. [H]

Amar Ibn al-Baytar: Z. Amar, "Ibn al-Baytar and the study of the plants of al-Sham", *Cathedra*, 76 (1995), pp. 49-76. [H].

Amar, Herbalist: Z. Amar, "Abu al-'abas al-Nabati – Andalusian herbalist in the Land of Israel in the Ayyubid Period", *Ariel*, 100-101 (1994), pp. 235-239. [H]

Amar, Innovations: Z. Amar, "Agronomic innovations as reflected in the commentary on sacred books and Jewish law in the Middle Ages", *BDD*, 3 (1996), pp. 87-97. [H]

Amar, Islam: Z. Amar, "Grape cultivation and wine production in Judea and Samaria during the Middle Ages", in: *Judea and Samaria Research Studies – Proceedings of the Fourth Conference,* Kedumim-Ariel 1995, pp. 247-261. [H]

Amar, Metamorphosis: Z. Amar, "The Metamorphosis of Holy Sites for Healin Purposes in Jerusalem", in: *Judea and Samaria Research Studies*, VII (Y. Eshel ed.), Tel-Aviv 1998, pp. 207-222. [H]

Amar, Preservation: Z. Amar, "The preservation of sacred healing sites in Jerusalem", in: *Judea and Samaria Research Studies – Proceedings of the Seventh Conference,* Kedumim-Ariel 1997, pp. 207-222. [H].

Amar, Theriac: Z. Amar, "The export of theriac from the Land of Israel and its uses in the Middle Ages", *Korot,* 12 (1996-1997), pp. 16-29. [H]

Amar, Traditions: Z. Amar, "Traditions and realia in the writing of a tenth century physician in Jerusalem" *Cathedra,* 81 (1996), pp. 23-34. [H]

Amundsen & Ferngren: D.W.Amundsen & G.B.Ferngren, "The Perception of Disease and Disease Causality in the New Testament", *Aufstieg und Niedergang der Romischen Welt* (ANRW), 37.3 (1996), pp. 2934-2956.

Amundsen: D.W. Amundsen, "The Medical Legislation of Assizes of Jerusalem", *Proceedings of the XXIII International Congress of the History of Medicine*, I, London 1974, pp. 517–522.

Antonini Placentini: Antonini Placentini, Itinerarium, P. Geyer (ed.), "Itineraria et alia geographica", *CCSL*, CLXXV, Tvrnholti 1965.

Arce: A. Arce, *Miscelanea de Tierra Santa*, I, Jerusalem 1950.

Arnold von Harff: E. von Groote, *Die Pilgerfahrt des Ritters Arnold von Harff*, Coln 1860.

Ashkenzai, Curing: Y. Ashkenazi, "Curing and Nursing in the Church of Jerusalem during the Byzantine Period" in: Z. Amar, E. Lev and J. Schwartz (eds.) *Medicine in Jerusalem throughout the Ages*. Tel-Aviv 1999. pp. 33-50. [H].

Ashkenzai, Involvement : Y. Ashkenazi, "Church involvement in medical services in Byzantine Eretz-Israel", in: *Illness and Healing in Ancient Times*, Haifa 1996. pp. 46-51.

Ashtor: E. Ashtor, "Jerusalem in the later Middle Ages", *Jerusalem: A Quarterly for the Research of Palestine*, II/2 (1955), pp. 71-116. [H]

Assaf: S.Assaf, *Beoholei Ya'akov*, Jerusalem 1965. [H]

Assises: A. Beugnot (ed.), "Les Assises de Jerusalem", *RHC,* Lois I–II, Paris 1841–1843.

Auld & Steiner: G.Auld & M.Steiner, *Jerusalem I*, Cambridge 1996.

Avigad & Sass: N.Avigad & B.Sass, *Corpus of West Semitic Stamp Seals*, Jerusalem 1997.

Avigad: N. Avigad, *The Upper City of Jerusalem*, Jerusalem 1980. [H].

Avoth de-Rabbi Nathan: Avoth de-Rabbi Nathan, Solomon Schechter Edition (M. Kister ed.), New-York - Jerusalem 1997.

Bagatti: B. Bagatti, "Father Anthony Manzazi of Cuna (1650–1729), Inventor of 'The Balm of Jerusalem'", *Franciscan Studied*, 6 (1946), pp. 250–361.

Bahat, Layout: D. Bahat, "The Physical Layout", in: *The History of Jerusalem: The Early Islamic Period* (638-1099) (J. Prawer ed.), Jerusalem 1987, pp. 32-79. [H]

Bahat, Proposal : D. Bahat, "A new proposal for dating the Medaba Map, *Ariel*, 116 (1996), pp. 74-75. [H]

Bahat, Topography: D. Bahat, "Topography and Archaeology", in: *The History of Jerusalem: Crusaders and Ayyubids (1099-1250)* (J. Prawer & H. Ben-Shammai ed.), Jerusalem 1991, pp. 68-134. [H]

Basola: I. Ben-Zvi, *A Pilgrimage to Palestine by Rabbi Moshe Basola of Ancona*, Jerusalem 1938. [H]

Behrens-Abousif: D. Behrens-Abouseif, *Fath Allah and Abu Zakariyya: Physicians under the Mamluks*, Cairo 1987.

Ben-Arieh: Y. Ben-Arieh, *A City Reflected in its Time*, Jerusalem 1977-1979. [H]

Benayahu, Generation: M. Benayahu, *A Single Generation in the Land*, Jerusalem 1988. [H]

Benayahu, Anthology: M. Benajahu, "Anthology of relationships of Land of Israel sages with the sages of Italy", *Sinai,* 35 (1954), pp. 55-66. [H]

Benayahu, Concerning: M. Benajahu, "Concerning medicine in an unknown manuscript of Rabbi Hayyim Vital", *Koroth* 9 (3-4): (1986) pp. 3-17. [H].

Benayahu, Extracts: M. Benayahu, "Extracts from the medicine and properties manuscript of Rabbi Hayyim Vital", *Korot* 9 (5-6): (1987) pp. 91-112. [H]

Benayahu, Jerusalem: M. Benayahu, "Rabbi Hayyim Vital in Jerusalem", *Sinai,* 30 (1952), pp. 65-75. [H]

Ben-Habib: Moshe Ben-Habib, *A Simple Bill of Divorce,* Jerusalem 1966. [H]

Benoit: P. Benoit, "Decouvertes archeologiques autour de la piscine de Bethesda", Jerusalem Through the Ages, The Twenty-fifth Archeological Convention, Jerusalem 1968, pp. 48-57.

Ben-Zvi: Y. Ben-Zvi, *The Land of Israel and its Settlement under Ottoman Rule,* Jerusalem 1976. [H]

Bergman: A. Bergman, *Bear Peace to the Mountains*, Jerusalem 1978. [H]

Bliss & Dickie: F.J. Bliss & A.C. Dickie, *Excavations at Jerusalem 1894-1897*, London 1898.

Boucher: J. Boucher, *Le Bouquet Sacre ou le voyage de la Terre Sainte*, Rouen 1752.

Brin: G.Brin, "On the Title: בן מלך", *Leshonenu*, 31 (1967), pp. 85-96. [H]
Burgoyne: M.H. Burgoyne, *Mamluk Jerusalem*, London 1987.
Cahen: C. Cahen, "Indigenes et Croises, Quelques mots a propos d'un medecin d'Amaury et de Salasin", *Syria*, 15 (1934), pp. 351–360.
Carpi:.D. Carpi, *Renaissance and Ghetto*, Tel-Aviv 1989.[H].
Carstens: H.R. Carstens, "The History of Hospitals with Special Reference to Some of the World's Oldest Institutions", *Annals of International Medicine,* 10 (1936), pp. 670–682.
Casola: M.M. Newett (ed.), *Canon Pietro Casola's Pilgrimage to Jerusalem in the Year 1494*, Manchester 1907.
Chapman: R.Chapman, "A Stone Toilet Seat Found in Jerusalem in 1925", *PEQ,* 124 (1992), pp. 4-8
Clark: K.W. Clark, *Checklist of Manuscripts in the Libraries of the Greek and Armenian Patriarchates in Jerusalem*, Washington 1953.
Cohen, Economy: A. Cohen, *Economic Life in Ottoman Jerusalem*, Cambridge 1989.
Cohen, 16 Century: A. Cohen & E. Simon-Pikali, *Jews in the Moslem Religious Court (in the XVIth Century)*, Jerusalem.[H]
Cohen, 18 Century: A. Cohen, E. Simon-Pikali & O. Salama, *Jews in the Moslem Religious Court (in the XVIIIth Century)*, Jerusalem 1996. [H]
Cohen, Jewish: A. Cohen, *The Jewish Community of Jerusalem in the 16th Century*, Jerusalem 1982. [H]
Conforote: D.Conforote, Kore Ha-Dorot (D. Cassel ed.), Berlin 1846.[H]
Conrad: L.I. Conrad, "Usama ibn Munqidh and Other Witnesses to Frankish and Islamic Medicine in the Era of the Crusades", In: Z. Amar, E. Lev & J. Schwartz (eds.), *Medicine in Jerusalem Throughout the Ages*, Tel Aviv 1999, pp. IXXX–LVI.
Cooley: R. Ya'akov Cooley, *Me'Am Loez Compilation,* Jerusalem 1969.
Crown: A.D.Crown, "The Knowledge of Drugs in Ancient Israel", *Australian Journal of Forensic Science*, 1970, pp. 30-48.
Custodia*:* *Custodia di Terra Santa 1342–1942*, Jerusalem 1951.
Dauphin: C. Dauphin, "Dora-Dor: A Pilgrim station on the way to Jerusalem", *Cathedra*, 29 (1983), pp. 29-44. [H]
David, Collections: A. David, Collections of the Institute of Microfilmed Hebrew Manuscripts, Jerusalem 1986. [H]
David, Immigration: A. David, *The Immigration and Settlement in the Land of Israel in the 16th Century*, Jerusalem 1993. [H].
David, Letter: A.David, "The Letter of R. Israel Ashkenazi of Jerusalem to Abraham of Perugia", *Alei-Sefer*, 16 (1990), pp, 95-122 . [H]
Davies: R.W.Davies, *Service in the Roman Army*, Edinburgh 1989.
Davis & Kloner: D.Davis & A.Kloner, "A Burial Cave of the Late Israelite Period on the Slopes of Mt. Zion", *Qadmoniot*, 41 (1978), pp. 16-19. [H]
Delaville: J. Delaville le Roulx, *Les Hospitalaris en Terre Sainte et a Chypre*, Paris 1904.
Dioscorides: R.T. Gunther (trans.), *The Greek Herbal of Dioscorides*, New–York 1959.
Dolev: E. Dolev, "The Saint Johns Hospital during the Crusader period in Jerusalem", *Harefua* 99 (1980), pp. 136-137. [H]
Downey: G. Downey, "Philanthropia in Religion and Statecraft in the Fourth Century after Christ", *Historia*, 4 (1955), pp. 199–208.
Droianov: A. Droianov, *From Early Days* II, Tel-Aviv 1935. [H]
Drory, Emir: J.Drory, The Emir Builder - The Story of Sayf al-Din Tankiz", *Zev Vilnay's Jubilee Volume*, II, Jerusalem 1987, pp. 195-204. [H]
Drory, Impact: J. Drory, "The Impact of the Mamluk's Rule on the History of Palestine", in: *Palestine in the Mamluk Period* (J. Drory ed.), Jerusalem 1992, pp. 1-12. [H]
Drory, Jerusalem: J. Drory, "Jerusalem in the Mamluk Period", in: *Jerusalem in the Middle Ages* (Z. Kedar ed.), Jerusalem 1979, pp. 148-184. [H]
Dubnov: S. Dubnov, "Jewish students at the university in Padua" in: *Sefer Hashanah: American Hebrew Year Book*, 1, 1931, pp. 216-219. [A]
Dvorjetski, Health: E. Dvorjetski, "Public Health in Jerusalem During the Second Temple Period, in: *Medicine in Jerusalem* (Z. Amar, E. Lev & J.Schwarts ed.), Tel-Aviv 1999, pp. 7-31. [H]
Dvorjetski, Springs: E. Dvorjetski, "Medicinal Hot Springs in Eretz-Israel in Antiquity - Sacred place or Popular sites of Healing?", *Jerusalem Studies in Jews Folklore*, 16 (1994), pp. 7-27. [H]
Edde: A.M. Edde, "Les Medecins dans la Societe Syrienne du VIIe/XIIIe siecle", *Annales Islamologiques*, 29 (1995), pp. 91–109.
Edelstein , Asclepius: E.J.Edelstein & L. Edelstein, *Asclepius: A Collection and Interpretation of the Testimonies*, II, Baltimore 1945, pp. 139-180.
Edelstein, Villa: G. Edelstein, "A Roman Villa at 'Ein Ya'el", *Qadmoniot*, 103-104 (1993), pp. 114-119. [H]
Eliav: M.Eliav, Eretz-Israel and its Yishuv in the 19th Century, Jerusalem 1978. [H]

Ell: S.R. Ell, "Pilgrims, Crusaders and Plagues", In: M. Waserman & S.S. Kottek (eds.), *Health and Disease in the Holy Land*, Lewiston–Queenston–Lampeter 1996, pp. 173–187.
Ernoul: Ernoul, "L'estat se la citez de Iherusalem", In: H. Michelant & G. Raynaud (eds.), *Itineraires a Jerusalem*, Geneve 1882.
Fahndrich: H. Fahndrich, *Treatise to Salah Ad–Din on the Revival of the Art of Medicine*, Wiesbaden 1983.
Farris & Storme: G. Farris & A. Storme, *Ceramica e Farmacia di San Salvatore a Gerusalemme*, Bologna 1981.
Ficarra: B.J. Ficarra, "Disease to Death during the Crusaders", In: M. Waserman & S.S. Kottek (eds.), *Health and Disease in the Holy Land*, Lewiston–Queenston–Lampeter 1996, pp. 135–155.
Fort: G.F. Fort, *Medical Economy during the Middle Ages*, New-York 1970.
Fraenkel, Endowing: Y. Fraenkel, The Endowing of the al-Madrasa al-Salahiyya Religious Foundation (Waqf) by Saladin, in: *Palestine in the Mamluk Period*, (J.Drory ed.) Jerusalem 1992, pp. 64-85.
Fraenkel, Establishment: Y.Frenkel, "The Establishment of the Waqf al-Hanaqah al- Sallahya by Sallah al-Din", *Cathedra*, 65 (1992), pp. 21-36. [H]
Freidin: I. Freidin, "Bikur Holim Perushim in Jerusalem", Cathedra, 27 (1983), pp. 117-140. [H]
Freiman: A. H. Freiman, "By-laws of Jerusalem", Book of Denburg, Jerusalem 1949, pp. 206-214. [H]
Friedenwald: H. Friedenwald, *The Jews and Medicine Essays*, Baltimore 1944.
Friedman, Eretz: Y. Friedman, "Eretz-Israel and Jerusalem on the eve of the Ottoman Period", in: Jerusalem in the Early Ottoman Period (A. Cohen ed.), Jerusalem 1979, pp. 7-38. [H]
Frumkin-Rivlin: A. L. Frumkin and A. Rivlin, *History of the Rabbinic Sages of Jerusalem,* Jerusalem, 1928-1933. [H]
Gabrieli: F. Gabrieli (trans.), *Arab Historians of the Crusades*, London 1969.
Gamil: Y. el-Gamil, "Karaite Jews in Egypt (1517-1918), in: *The Jews in Ottoman Egypt* (1517-1914)", (J.M.Landau ed.), Jerusalem 1988, pp. 513-556. [H]
Gat: B. Gat, "The first medical institution in Eretz-Israel", *Yerushalayim: Review for Eretz-Israel Research*, 1 (1953), pp. 259-272 [H].
Gayger: Y. Gayger, "The spread of Christianity in the land of Israel from its inception until the days of Julian" in: *Eretz-Israel from the Destruction of the Second Temple until the Muslim Conquest* (Z. Baras, S.Safrai, M.Stern & Y. Tsafrir eds.), Jerusalem 1982, pp. 218-233. [H]
Gelber: N.M. Gelber, "On the history of Jewish doctors in 18th century Poland" in: *Tribute to Yeshayahu* (Y. Tirosh, ed.), Tel-Aviv 1957, pp. 347-371. [H]
Germer-Durand: J. Germer-Durand, "Epigraphie Chretienne de Jerusalem", *Revue Biblique*, 1 (1892), pp. 560–588.
Gersht: R. Gersht, "Gods of Medicine in the Greek and Roman World", in: *Illness and Healing in Ancient Time* (O. Rimon ed), Haifa 1996, pp. 8-12.
Gichon & Isaac: M. Gichon and B.H. Isaac, "A Flavian Inscription from Jerusalem", *IEJ*, 24 (1974), pp. 117-123.
Gil: M. Gil, *Palestine during the First Muslim Period (643-1099),* Tel-Aviv 1983. [H]
Goitein Jewry: S.D. Goitein, *Palestinian Jewry in Early Islamic and Crusader Times*, Jerusalem 1980. [H]
Goitein Society: S.D. Goitein, *A Mediterranean Society*, Berkeley 1967–1988.
Grajewsky: P. Ben Zvi Grajewsky, *From Ancient Archives*, Jerusalem 1977. [H]
Green & Tsafrir: J.Green & Y.Tsafrir, "Greek Inscriptions from Hammat-Gader: A Poem by the Empress Eudocia and Two Building Inscriptions", *Qadmoniot*, 61 (1983), pp. 28-36. [H]
Greenbaum:A. Greenbaum, *The Biblical Commentary of Rav Samuel ben Hofni Gaon*, Jerusalem 1978. [H]
Griffith: S.H.Griffith, "Holy Land history from the archive of old South Palestinian Arabic texts", *Cathedra*, 69 (1993), pp. 57-78. [H]
Hacker, Connections: J. Hacker, "The Connections of Spanish Jewry with Eretz-Israel between 1391 and 1492", *Shalem*, 1 (1974), pp. 105-156.
Hacker, Elija: J. Hacker, "R. Elija of Massa Lombarda in Jerusalem", *Zion,* 50 (1985), pp. 241-263. [H]
Haggai: S. Haggai, "Early physicians and medicine in the land of Israel", *Mahanaim* 77(1963) pp. 82-87. [H]
Hajiz, Commandments: R. Moshe Hajiz, *The Book of Commandments,* Parmisla 1913. [H]
Hajiz, Halachot: R. Ya'akov Hajiz, *The Book of Halachot Ktanot*, Venice 1704. [H]
Halevi: S. Halevi, *Early Episodes in the History of the Yishuv,* 1989 pub. site not noted). [H]
Hamarneh, Development: S. Hamarneh, "Development of Hospitals in Islam", *Journal of the History of Medicine and Allied Sciences*, 17 (1962), pp. 366– 384.
Har-El: M. Har-El, "Water for Purification, Hygiene and Cult at the Temple in Jerusalem", *Eretz-Israel*, 19 (1987), pp. 310-313.[H]
Hasselquist: F. Hasselquist, *Voyages and Travels in the Levant*, London 1866. (The original text was published as F. Hasselquist, *Iter Palaestinum*, Stockholm 1757)
Hasson: I. Hasson, "Remarrues sur l'inscription de l'epoque de Mu'awiya a Hammat Gader", *IEJ*, 32 (182), pp. 97–101.
Heyd, History: W. Heyd, *Histoire du Commerce du Levant au Moyen–Age*, Leipzig 1936.
Heyd, Moses: U. Heyd, "Moses Hamon, Chief Jewish Physician to Sultan Suleyman the Magnificent", *Oriens*, 16 (1963), pp. 152–170.

Heyd, Documents: U. Heyd, *Ottoman Documents on Palestine 1552-1615*, Oxford 1960.
Heyd, Jews: U.Heyd, "The Jews of Eretz-Israel in the Late Seventeenth Century", Yerushalayim*: Review for Eretz-Israel Research*, 1 (1953), pp. 173-184.
Hirschfeld, Hammat: Y. Hirschfeld, *The Roman Baths of Hammat Gader*, Jerusalem 1997.
Hirschfeld, Monasteries: Y.Hirschfeld, The Judean desert monasteries in the Byzantine Period Ph.D Thesis, Jerusalem 1987. [H]
Hogan: L. Hogan, "Healing in the Second Temple Period", Thesis for the degree of Doctor of Philosophy, Jerusalem 1986.
Holum: K.G. Holum, *Theodosian Empressed*, Berkeley–Los Angeles–London 1982.
Horn: E. Horn, *Ichnographiae Monumentorum Terrae Sanctae*, E. Hoade & B. Bagatti (eds.), Jerusalem 1962.
Hospitalier documents: J. Delaville le Roulx (ed.), *Cartulaire General de L'ordre des Hospitaliers de S. Jean de Jerusalem, 1100–1310*, Paris 1894–1906.
Hume: E.E. Hume, *Medical Work of the Knights Hospitallers of Saint John of Jerusalem*, Baltimore 1940.
Ibn abi Usaybi'a: Ibn abi Usaybi'a, 'Ahmad ibn al-Qasim, *'Uyun al-'anba' fi tabaqat al-'atibba'*, ed. N. Rida, Beirut 1965. [A]
Ibn al-Aṯir, al-Kamil: 'Ibn al-'Aṯir, 'Izz al-Din 'Ali ibn Muhammad, *al-Kamil fi al-tarikh*, Beirut 1966-1967. [A]
Ibn al-Aṯir, al-Lubab: 'Ibn al-'Aṯir, 'Izz al-Din 'Ali ibn Muhammad, *al-Lubab fi tahḏib al-'ansab*, Beirut n.d.. [A]
Ibn al-Qifti: 'Ibn al-Qifti, 'Ali ibn Yusuf, *Tarikh al-hukama'*, ed. J. Lippert, Leipzig 1903. [A]
Ibn Jubayr: Ibn Jubayr, Muhammad ibn Ahmad, *al-Rihla*, ed. De Goeje (revised ed. A. R. Gibb Hamilton), Leiden 1907. [A]
Ibn Kaṯir: Ibn Kaṯir, Isma'il ibn 'Amr, *al-Bidaya wa-al-nihaya*, Beirut 1977. [A]
Ibn Khaldun: Ibn Khaldun, The Muqaddimah (F. Rosenthal trans.), III, London 1958 [A]
Ibn Munqid: 'Ibn Munqid, 'Usama ibn Muršid, *Kitab al-'i'tibar*, ed. P. K. Hitti, Princeton 1930. [A]
Ibn Qadi: 'Ibn Qadi Šuhba, 'Abu Bakr ibn 'Ahmad, *Tarikh Ibn Qadi Šuhba*, ed. A. Darwiš, I, Damascus 1977. [A]
Isaacs: H. Isaacs, "The Impact of Western Medicine on Muslim Physicians and their Writing in the 17th Century", *Bulletin of the British Association of Orientalists*, 11 (1979–1980), pp. 52–57.
'Isa, Tarikh: A. 'Isa, *Tarikh al-bimaristanat fi al-'islam*, Damascus 1939.
'Isa, Dictionary: A. 'Isa, *Dictionnaire des Noms des Plantes*, Cairo 1930.
Jadon, Comparison: S. Jadon, "A Comparison of the Wealth, Prestige, and Medical Work of the Physicians of Salah al-Din in Egypt and Syria", *Bulletin of the History of Medicine*, 44 (1970), pp. 64–75.
Jadon, Physicians: S. Jadon, "The Physicians of Syria during the Reign of Salah al-Din 570–589 A.H. 1174–1193 A.D.", *Journal of the History of Medicine and Allied Sciences*, 25 (1970), pp. 323–340.
Jeffers: A. Jeffers, *Magic and Divination in Ancient Palestine and Syria*, Leiden New-York Koln
Joannes Moschus: Joannes Moschus, Pratum spirituale, *PG*, 87 (3), pp. 2847–3116.
Jones: A.H.M. Jones, *The Greek City*, Oxford 1940.
Josephus, JA: Josephus, Jewish Antiquities (R.Marcus tran.), London 1966
Josephus, JW: Josephus, The Jewish War (H.J.Thackeray tran.), London 1967
Joshua: Y. Joshua, "Some information on the Jews of Jerusalem during the Turkish period", Sinai 76 (1975) pp, 275-279. [H]
Kafih: J. Kafih, *Rabbi Sa'adia Gaon's Commentary on the Torah*, Jerusalem 1984. [H]
Kaplan: J. Kaplan, "Jewish Students of Leyden University in the 17th Century", Studies on the History of Dutch Jewry, 2 (1979), pp. 65-75.[H]
Kass: A.M. Kass, "Western Medicine in Nineteenth-Century Jerusalem", *Journal of the History of Medicine and Allied Sciences,* 44 (1989), pp. 447–461.
Kedar Benvenutus: B.Z. Kedar, "Benvenutus Grpheus of Jerusalem, an Oculist in the Era of the Crusades", *Korot*, 11 (1995), pp. 14–41.
Kedar hospital: B.Z. Kedar, "A Twelfth-Century Description of the Jerusalem Hospital", In: H. Nicholson (ed.) *The Military Orders, II, Welfare and Warfare,* Aldershot 1998, pp. 3–26.
Kee: H.C.Kee, Medicine, Miracle and Magic in New Testament Time, Cambridge 1986, pp. 88-94.
Khusraw: Khusraw, Nasir, *Sefer nameh*, ed. & trans. C. Schefer, Paris 1881 (repr. Amsterdam 1970). [A]
Kings: E.J. King, *The Knights Hospitallers in the Holy Land*, London 1931.
Klein-Franke: F. Klein-Franke, "Health and Healing in Medieval Muslim Palestine", In: M. Waserman & S.S. Kottek (eds.), *Health and Disease in the Holy Land*, Lewiston–Queenston–Lampeter 1996, pp. 103–134.
Kohlberg & Kedar: E. Kohlberg & B.Z. Kedar, "A Melkite Physician in Frankish Jerusalem and Ayyubid Damascus: Muwaffaq al-Din Yaqub b. Siqlab", *Asian and African Studies*, 22 (1988), pp. 113–126.
Koren: N.Koren, *Jewish Physicians: A Biographical Index*, Jerusalem 1973.
Kottek: S.S. Kottek, *Medicine and Hygiene in the Works of Flavius Josephus*, Leiden-New-York-Koln 1994.
Kroyanker: D. Kroyanker, *City Hall Complex*, Jerusalem 1993. [H]
Kupfer: E.Kupfer, "The Jewish Community of Safed and the Activity of R. Menahem Azariah of Fano on Behalf of the Yishuv in Eretz-Israel", *Shalem*, 2 (1976), pp. 361- 364.

Lazare's documents: A. De Marsy, "Fragment d'un cartulaire de l'ordre de Saint-Lazare, en Terre Sainte", *Archives de L'Orient Latin*, 2 (1884), pp. 121–158.

Leclerc, History: L. Leclerc, *Histoire de la medecine arabe*, New–York 1971.

Leibowitz: J.O. Leibowitz *Encyclopaedia Biblica*, VII, Jerusalem 1976.,

Leibowitz: Y. Leibowitz, "On the history of Jewish hospitals in Jerusalem", *Assia,* 6 (1978), pp. 26-30. [H]

Levinger: Y. Levinger, "Forbidden types of work and the reasons according to Maimonides", *Jerusalem Studies in Jewish Thought,* 2 (1983), pp. 515-528. [H]

Levy, History: N. Levy, *The History of Medicine in the Holy Land: 1799-1948*, Tel-Aviv 1998. [H]

Levy, Maps: M. Levy, "Medieval Maps of Jerusalem", in: *The History of Jerusalem: Crusaders and Ayyubids (1099-1250),* (J.Prawer & H. Ben-Shammai ed.), Jerusalem 1991, pp. 418-507. [H]

Lewis Maimonides: B. Lewis, "Maimonides, Lionheart, and Saladin", *Eretz–Israel*, 7 (1964), pp. 70–75.

Lewis: B. Lewis, *On History (Collected Studies)*, Jerusalem 1988.

Lieberman: S. Lieberman, *Greek and Hellenism in Jewish Palestine*, Jerusalem 1991. [H]

Limor: O.Limor, *Holy Land Travels*, Jerusalem 1998. [H]

Little, Catalogue: D.P. Little, *A Catalogue of the Islamic Documents from al–Haram al–Sharif in Jerusalem*, Beirut 1984.

Little, Significance: D.P. Little, "The Significance of the Haram Documents for the Study of Medieval Islamic History", *Der Islam*, 57 (1980), pp. 189–219.

Little, Documents: D. P. Little, "Haram Documents Related to the Jews of Late Fourteenth-Century Jerusalem", in: Palestine in the Mamluk Period (J. Drory ed.), Jerusalem 1992, pp.189-219. [H]

Luncz: A.M. Luncz, "Superstitions*", Jerusalem,* 1 (1881), pp. 20-28. [H]

Lutfi: H. Lutfi, *al–Quds al–Mamlukiyya*, Berlin 1985.

Macalister: R.A.S. Macalister, "The Rock-cut Tombs in Wady er-Rababi, Jerusalem", *PEFQS* (1900), pp. 225–248.

Maimonides Glossaire: Moshe Ben Maimon (Maimonides*), Un Glossaire de Matiere Medicale Compose par Maimonide* (M. Meyerhof, ed.) *Memoires Presentes a l'Institut d'Egypte*, 41 (1940).

Maimonides Poisons: Moshe Ben Maimon*, Poisons and their Antidotes* (S. Muntner, ed.), Jerusalem 1942. [H]

Maimonides, Aphorisms: Moshe Ben Maimon, *Aphorisms of Moses* (S. Muntner ed.), Jerusalem 1961. [H]

Maimonides, Asthma: Moshe Ben Maimon, *On Asthma* (S. Muntner ed.), Jerusalem 1965. [H]

Maimonides, Mishna: Moshe Ben Maimon, *Mishna with commentary of Rabbi Moshe Ben Maimon,* (Y. Kafih ed.), Jerusalem 1963-1967. [H]

Maimonides, Regimen: Moshe Ben Maimon, *Regimen Sanitatis* (S. Muntner ed.), Jerusalem 1957. [H]

Malki: M. Benayahu. *Medical Works of Rabbi Refael Mordecai Malki* , Jerusalem 1985. [H]

Mann: J. Mann, *Texts and Studies in Jewish History and Literature*, II, Philadelphia 1935.

Margalit, Ramban: D. Margalit, "The Ramban (Nachmanides, 1194-1270) as a physician", *Koroth* 1(9-10) (1956) pp. 303-315.[H].

Margalit, Way:. Margalit, *The Way of Israel in Medicine*, Jerusalem 1970. [H]

Mazar, Camp: E. Mazar, "The camp of the Tenth Roman Legion at the foot of the south-west corner of the Temple Mount enclosure wall in Jerusalem", in: *New Studies on Jerusalem, Proceedings of the Fifth Conference* (A.Faust & E.Baruch eds.), Ramat-Gan 1999, p. 52-67 [H]

Mazar, Survey: A. Mazar, "A survey of the aqueducts leading to Jerusalem", in: *The Aqueducts of Ancient Palestine* (D. Amit, Y. Hirschfeld & J. Patrich ed.), Jerusalem 1989, pp. 169-195. [H]

Mazor & Bar-Natan: G. Mazor and R. Bar-Natan, "Public Hygiene and Baths in Nysa Scythopolis", *Michmanim*, 13 (1999), pp. 59-72. [H]

Mechilta D'Rabbi Ismael: H.S.Horovitz & I.A.Rabin, *Mechilta D'Rabbi Ismael*, Jerusalem 1970. [H]

Melanie: D. Gorce, *Vie de Sainte Melanie*, Paris 1962.

Mendelsohn: I.Mendelsohn, "Guilds in Ancient Palestine", *BASOR*, 80 (1940), pp. 17-21.

Meshorer ,Coinage: Y. Meshorer, *The Coinage of Aelia Capitolina*, Jerusalem 1989.

Meshorer, Hygieia: Y.Meshorer, "Hygieia in Aelia Capitolina", *The Israel Museum Journal*, 1 (1982), pp. 17-18.

Meyerhof: M. Meyerhof, "Sultan Saladin's physician on the transmission of Greek medicine to the Arabs", *Bulletin of the History of Medicine*, 18 (1945), pp. 169–178.

Milik: J.T. Milik, "La topographie de Jerusalem vers la fin de l'epoque byzantine", *Melanges de l'Universite Saint–Joseph*, 37 (1961), pp. 127–189.

Miller, Birth: T.S. Miller, *The Birth of the Hospital in the Byzantine Empire*, Baltimore and London 1985.

Miller, Knights: T.S. Miller, "The knights of Saint John and the Hospitals of the Latin West", *Speculum*, 53 (1978), pp. 709–733.

Mizrachi: Rabbi Nissim Hayyim ben R. Moshe Mizrachi, *Sefer Admat Kodesh*, I-II, Constantinople 1742. [H]

Morgenstern: A. Morgenstern, "The first Jewish hospital in Jerusalem", *Cathedra*, 33 (1984), pp. 107-124. [H]

Morris: J.F. Morris, *The Penguin Book of the Middle Ages*, 1971.

Motzkin: A.L. Motzkin, "A thirteenth-century Jewish physician in Jerusalem", *Muslim World*, 60 (1970), pp. 344–349.

Mujir al-Din: Mujir al-Din, 'Abd al-Rahman ibn Muhammad, *al-'Uns al-jalil bi-tarikh al-Quds wa-al-Khalil*, Amman 1973.[A]

Murad: 'Ibrahim ibn Murad, *Buhuṯ fi tarikh al-tibb wa-al-saydala 'ind al-'arab*, Beirut 1991. [A]

Murphey: R.Murphey, "Ottoman medicine and transculturalism from the sixteenth through the eighteenth century", *Bulletin of the History of Medicine*, 66 (1992), pp. 376-403.

Nahamias: B.Nahmias, *Hamsa.* Tel-Aviv 1996. [H]

Neufeld: E.Neufeld, "Hygiene conditions in ancient Israel (Iron Age)", *Journal of the History of Medicine*, 25 (1970), pp. 414-437.

Neumann Medicine: B. Neumann, *Die Heillig Stadt und deren Bewohner,* Hamburg 1877, pp. 466–512.

Nilsson & Sunzel: I. Nilsson & H. Sunzel, "The influence of Medieval Christian ideology on western hospitals; medical care at the Hospitallers in Jerusalem", *Lychnos*, 1992, pp. 9–24.

Omar: R. Omar, "Full of health and poison; Popular use of the fig", *Teva Va'aretz,* 30 (1988), pp. 14-15. [H]

Ovadiah & de Silva: A. Ovadiah & C.G. de Silva, *Supplementum to the Corpus of the Byzantine Churches in the Holy Land,* Jerusalem 1984.

Ovadiah, Church: A.Ovadiah, "A Crusader Church in the Jewish Quarter of Jerusalem", *Eretz-Israel*, 11 (1973), pp. 208-212.[H]

Ovadiah, Corpus: A. Ovadiah, *Corpus of the Byzantine Churches in the Holy Land*, Bonn 1970.

Palmer: R. Palmer, "Pharmacy in the Republic of Venice in Sixteenth Century", In: A. Wear, R.K. French & I.M. Lonie (eds.), *The Medical Renaissance of the Sixteenth Century*, Cambridge 1985, pp. 100–117.

Parmentier: M.Parmentier, "The lasting sanctity of Bethesda", in: *Sanctity of Time and Space in Tradition and Modernity* (A.Houtman, M.J.H.M.Ppprthuis & J.Schwartz eds), Leiden - Boston - Koln 1998, pp. 73-93

Patai: Y. Patai, The Water, Tel-Aviv, 1936. [H]

Patrich, Monasticism: J.Patrich, The Judean desert monasticism in the Byzantine Period, Jerusalem 1985. [H]

Patrich, Structure: J. Patrich, "The structure of the Muristan Quarter of Jerusalem in the Crusader Period", *Cathedra*, 33 (1984), pp. 3-16. [H]

Piccirillo: M. Piccirillo, "The Umayyad Churches of Jordan", *ADAJ*, 28 (1984), pp. 333–341.

Plessner: M.Plessner, "On Daud al-Antaki's Medical and Magical Encyclopaedia and some of its Sources", *Eretz-Israel*, 7 (1964), pp. 138-141. [H]

Prawer, Colonial: J. Prawer, *The Crusaders - A Colonial Society*, Jerusalem 1985. [H].

Prawer, Institutions: J. Prawer, *Crusader Institutions*, Oxford 1980.

Prawer, Epigraphy: J. Prawer, "Crusader Epigraphy in Jerusalem", in: The History of Jerusalem: Crusaders and Ayyubids (1099-1250), (J. Prawer & H. Ben-Shammai ed.), Jerusalem 1991, pp. 374-387. [H]

Prawer, Geo-Ethnography: J. Prawer, "Geo-Ethnography of Crusader Jerusalem", in: The History of Jerusalem: Crusaders and Ayyubids (1099-1250), (J. Prawer & H. Ben-Shammai ed.), Jerusalem 1991, pp. 135-149. [H]

Prawer, History: J. Prawer (ed.), The History of Eretz Israel under Moslem and Crusader Rule (634-1291), Jerusalem 1981.

Prawer, Jerusalem: J.Prawer, "Political History of Crusader and Ayyubid Jerusalem", in: *The History of Jerusalem: Crusaders and Ayyubids (1099-1250*), (J. Prawer & H. Ben-Shammai ed.), Jerusalem 1991, pp. 1-67. [H]

Prawer, Kingdom: J. Prawer, *A History of the Latin Kingdom of Jerusalem*, Jerusalem 1947. [H]

Preuss: J. Preuss, *Biblical and Talmudic Medicine*, F. Rosner (trans.), New-York 1983.

Pri Hadass: R. David De-Silva, ***Pri Hadass,*** mss. Zvi Malachi, no. 1, Institute of Hebrew Microfilmed Manuscripts at the National Library in Jerusalem, no. 38766. [H]

Price: R.M. Price (trans.), *Lives of the Monks of Palestine by Cyril of Scythopolis*, Michigan 1991.

Procopius: H.B. Dewing, *Procopius of Caesarea (LCL)*, London 1960.

Raba: J. Raba, *Russian Travel Accounts on Palestine*, Jerusalem 1986. [H]

Radbaz: Rabbi David ben Shlomo Ibn Zimra, *Responsa of the Radbaz*, Warsaw 1982. [H]

Rahmani: L.Y.Rahmani, *A Catalogue of Jewish Ossuaries in the Collections of the State of Israel*, Jerusalem 1994.

Ralbah: R. Levi Ibn Habib, *Responsa from the Ralbah*, Lemberg 1864 (new ed. Brooklyn 1962). [H]

Rauwolf: L. Rauwolf, *Aigentliche Beschreibung der Raiss inn die Morglenlaender,* Graz 1971. (facsimile of 1583 edition).

Reich & Billig: R. Reich & Y. Billig, "Theatre-Seats from the Excavations near the Temple Mount", in*: New Studies on Jerusalem, Proceedings of the Fifth Conference* (A.Faust & E.Baruch ed.), Ramat-Gan 1999, pp. 37-42 [H]

Reinhard & Warnock: K.Reinhard & P.Warnock, "Archaeoparasitology and analysis of the latrine pit soils from the City of David", in: *Illness and Healing in Ancient Time* (O.Rimon ed), Haifa 1996, pp. 20-23.

Reiss: N. Reiss, *The Health Care of the Arabs in Israel*, Boulder, San Francisco and Oxford 1991.

Richard. Hospitals: J. Richard, "Hospitals and Hospital Congregations in the Latin Kingdom during the First Period of the Frankish Conquest", In: B.Z. Kedar, H.E. Mayer & R.C. Smail (eds.), *Outremer,* Jerusalem 1982, pp. 89–100.

Richards, Jerusalem: D.S. Richards, "Saladin's Hospital in Jerusalem: Its Foundation and Some Later Archival Material", In: K. Athamina & R. Heacock (ed.), *The Frankish Wars and Their Influence on Palestine,* Birzeit 1994, pp. 70–83.

Riley-Smith: J. Riley-Smith, *The Knights of St. John in Jerusalem and Cyprus c.1050–1310*, London 1967.

Rimon: O. Rimon (ed.), 'Purity broke out in Israel' - Stone Vessels in the Late Second Temple Period, Haifa 1994.

Rivlin, Anthology: A.B. Rivlin, *Anthology of Commentary on the Pentateuch by Rephael Mordekhai Malki*, II, Jerusalem 1928. [H]

Rivlin, Thousand: Y. Y. Rivlin, *A Thousand and One Nights*, IV, Jerusalem 1961. [H]

Roger: F.E. Roger, *La Terre Sainte, ou Description topographique tres particuliere des Saints Lieux & de la Terre Promission*, Paris 1664.

Rohricht, Articles: R. Rohricht (ed.), *Beitrage zur Geschichte der Kreuzzuge*, Berlin 1878.

Rohricht, Regesta: R. Rohricht, *Regesta Regni Hierosolymitani and Additamentum*, Innsbruc 1893–1904.

Rose: R. Rose, "Communities of Eastern Christians in Crusader Jerusalem", in: *The History of Jerusalem: Crusaders and Ayyubids (1099-1250)* (J. Prawer & H. Ben-Shammai ed.), Jerusalem 1991, pp. 176-193.[H]

Rozen & Vitztum: M. Rozen & A. Vitztum, "The dark mirror of the soul- The dreams of a Jewish physician in Jerusalem in the late 17th century", *Simon Simonsohn Jubilee Volume*, Tel-Aviv 1993, p. 73-104. [H]

Rozen, Community: M.Rozen, *The Jewish Community of Jerusalem in the Seventeenth Century*, Tel-Aviv 1984.[H]

Rozen, Identity: M. Rozen, *Jewish Identity and Society in the Seventeenth Century: Reflections on the Life and Work of Refael Mordekhai Malki*, Tubingen 1992.

Rozen, Ruins: M.Rozen, *The Ruins of Jerusalem*, Tel-Aviv 1981.[H]

Ruderman: D.B. Ruderman, *Jewish Thought and Scientific Discovery in Early Modern Europe*, New Haven and London 1995.

Safrai, Pligrimage: S.Safrai, Pligrimage at the Time of the Second Temple, Tel-Aviv 1965 .[H]

Safrai, Sanctity: Z. Safrai, The Sanctity of Jerusalem in Desolation, in: *International Rennert Guest Lecture Series*, 4 (1999), pp. 1-45.[H]

Salama & Zilberman: O.Salama & Y.Zilberman, "Jerusalem's Water Supply in the 16th and 17th Centuries", *Cathedra*, 41 (1986), pp. 91-106. [H]

Sandoli: S. De Sandoli, *Itinera Hierosolymitana Crucesignatorum* (saec. XII–XIII), I–II, Jerusalem 1978–1980.

Schein: S. Schein, "Latin Aid Institutions in Ayyubid and Mamluk Jerusalem", in: *Palestine in the Mamluk Period,* (J.Drory ed.) Jerusalem 1992, pp. 142-156.

Schick, Christian: R. Schick, "Christian Life in Palestine during the Early Islamic Period", *Biblical Archaeologist*, 51 (1988), pp. 218–221, 239–240.

Schick, Communities: R. Schick, *The Christian Communities of Palestine from Byzantine to Islamic Rule*, Princeton New Jersey 1995.

Schick et al: C. Schick, C.W.W. Wilson & A.G.R. Conder, "Pool of Bethesda", *PEFQS*, 1888, pp. 111–134.

Schittny: H.R. Schittny, "Die historische Apotheke der Franziskaner in Jerusalem, *Geschichte der Pharmazie*, 45 (1993), pp. 41–45.

Scholem: G.Scholem, "Life and Works of R. Jacob Zemah", Kiryat Sefer, 26 (1950), pp. 185-194. [H]

Schur, Community: N. Schur, "The Jewish Community of Jerusalem in the 16th-18th Centuries According to Christian Chronicles and Travel Description", in: *Jerusalem in the Early Ottoman Period* (A. Cohen ed.), Jerusalem 1979, pp. 343-434.[H]

Schur, Franciscan: N. Schur, "Franciscan Physicians and Pharmacists in Jerusalem" in: Z. Amar, E. Lev and J. Schwartz (eds.) *Medicine in Jerusalem throughout the Ages*. Tel-Aviv 1999. pp. 99-106. [H]

Schur, History: N.Schur, *History of Jerusalem*, III, Tel-Aviv 1987.[H]

Schur, Voyage: N. Schur, *Voyage into the Past*, Jerusalem 1998.[H]

Schwake, Development: N. Schwake, *Die Entwicklug des Krankenhauswesns der Stadt Jerusalem von ende des 18 bis zum Beginn des 20 Jahrhunderts*, Herzogenrath 1983.

Schwake, Hospitals: N. Schwake, "Hospitals and European Colonial Policies in the 19th and Early 20th Centuries", In: M. Waserman & S.S. Kottek (eds.), *Health and Disease in the Holy Land*, Lewiston–Queenston–Lampeter 1996, pp. 231–262.

Schwartz: E. Schwartz, *Kyrillos Von Skythopolis*, Leipzig 1939.

Seetzen: U.J. Seetzen, *Reisen durch Syrien, Palestina etc.* II, Berlin 1854.

Segal: B.Z. Segal, *Geography in the Mishna*, Jerusalem 1979. [H]

Seide: J. Seide, "Medicine and Natural History in the Itinerary of Rabbi Benjamin of Tudela (1100–1177)", *Bulletin of the History of Medicine*, 5 (1954), pp. 401–407.

Seidler: E. Seidler, "Medieval Western Hospital: Social or Health Care Facilities?" In: Y. Kawakita et al. (eds.), *History of Hospitals – The Evolution of Health Care Facilities,* Tokyo 1986, pp. 5–22.

Sethune: M. Sethune, Book of Congregation for God's Name, Jerusalem 1874.[H]

Shachar, Seal: I. Shachar, "The Seal of Nahmanides", in: *Jerusalem in the Middle Ages* (Z. Kedar ed.), Jerusalem 1979, pp. 137-147.[H]

Shahar Lepers: S. Shahar, "Des Lepreux pas comme les autres, L'ordre de Saint-Lasare dans le royaume latin de Jerusalem", *Revue Historique*, 541 (1982), pp. 19–41.
Shahar, Groups: S. Shahar, *Marginal Groups in the Middle Ages*, Tel-Aviv 1985. [H]
Shiloh: Y.Shiloh, "A Hoard of Hebrew Bullae from the City of Jerusalem", *Eretz-Israel*, 18 (1985), pp. 73-87.[H].
Shoham: Y. Shoham, "Hebrew Bullae from the City of David", *Eretz-Israel*, 26 (1999), pp. 151-175.[H]
Shulvass: M.A.Shulvass, Rome and Jerusalem, Jerusalem 1944.[H]
Shvartz, Grains: Y. Shvartz, *The Grains of the Land*, Jerusalem 1900. [H]
Shvartz: S. Shvartz, "Ethnicity, religion, and politics in establishing Jewish medical institutions in 19th century Jerusalem", *Korot*, 9 (1989), pp. 232-242. [H]
Sibt ibn al-Jawzi: Sibt ibn al-Jawzi, Yusufl, *Mir'at al-zaman fi tarikh al-'a'yan*, 8a, Hyderabad 1951. [A]
Singer: A. Singer, "Ottoman Palestine (1516–1800): Health, Disease, and Historical Source", In: M. Waserman & S.S. Kottek (eds.),*Health and Disease in the Holy Land*, Lewiston–Queenston–Lampeter 1996, pp. 189–206.
Slushatz: N. Slushatz, "The yishuv in the land of Israel and Syria in the 16th century", *Society for the Study of Eretz-Israel and its Antiquities,* 3 (1935), pp. 323-338. [H]
Smith, Jesus: M. Smith, Jesus the Magician, New-York - London 1978
Smith, Science: A.G.R. Smith, *Science and Society in the Sixteenth and Seventeenth Centuries*, London 1972.
Sohastov: G. Sohastov, *Sacred Monument*, Lemberg, 1863-1865. [H]
Stern, Encyclopedia: E. Stern (ed.), *The New Encyclopedia of Archaeological Excavations in the Holy Land*, IV, Jerusalem 1992, p. 1483.
Stern: S. Stern, "The First Jewish Hospital in Jerusalem - An Addendum", *Cathedra*, 37 (1985), pp. 184-188.[H]
Sterns: I. Sterns, "Care of the Sick Brothers by the Crusader Orders in the Holy Land", *Bulletin of the History of Medicine*, 57 (1983), pp. 43–69.
Stiebel: G.D.Stiebel, "The Whereabouts of the Xth Legion and Boundaries of Aelia Capitolina", in: *New Studies on Jerusalem, Proceedings of the Fifth Conference* (A.Faust & E.Baruch ed.), Ramat-Gan 1999, pp. 74-75 [H]
Strauss: A. Strauss (Ashtor), *The History of the Jews in Egypt and Syria*, Tel-Aviv, 1951. [H]
Strehlke: E. Strehlke (ed.), *Tabulae Ordinis Theutonici*, Berlin 1869; Photo. reprint with an introduction by H.E. Mayer, Toronto 1975.
Tamimi: al-Tamimi, *al-Mursid ila Jawahir al-Aghdhiya wa-Quwa al-Mufradat min al-Adwiya*, MS Paris, Bibliotheque Nationale, no. 2870. [A]
Templars Rule: J.M. Upton–Ward (trans.), The Rule of the Templars, Burg St. Edmonds 1992.
Theodosios: H. Usener (ed.), *Der Heilige Theodosios*, Leipzig 1890.
Theophrastus: Theophrastus, *Enquiry into Plants* (A.Hort tran.), London 1980 (LCL)
Tobler, Medicine: T. Tobler, *Beitrag zur medizinischen Topographie von Jerusalem*, Berlin 1855.
Toledano: Toledano, Y.M. *Light of the West*, Jerusalem, 1989.[H]
Tosephta: M.S. Zuckermandel ed., *Tosephta*, Jerusalem 1970.[H]
Treatise Semahot: *Treatise Semahot (*M. Higger ed.), New-York 1931.
Tsafrir, Eretz Israel: Y. Tsafrir, *Eretz Israel from the Destruction of the Second Temple to the Muslim Conquest*, II, Jerusalem 1984.[H]
Tsafrir, Zion: Y. Tsafrir, "Zion – The south-western hill of Jerusalem and its place in the urban development of the city in the Byzantine Period", Thesis submitted for the degree of Doctor of Philosophy, Jerusalem 1975. [H]
Tuito: D. Tuito, "Rabbi Hezekiah De Silva; His mission, books, and teaching" in: *Tribute to Abraham* (A. Berger ed.), Jerusalem 1986, pp. 53-75. [H]
Ulman, Plants: S. B. Ulman, "Medicinal plants in the Bible", *Sinai,* 26 (1950), pp. 194-205. [H]
Vetrali: L. Vetrali, "Le iscrizioni dell acquedotto Romano presso Betlemme", *Studii Biblici Franciscani Liber Annuus*, 17 (1967), pp. 149-161.
Vilnay: Z. Vilnay, *Jerusalem, Capital of Israel, IV,* Jerusalem 1971. [H]
Vincent & Abel: L.H. Vincent & F.M. Abel, *Jerusalem nouvelle*, II, Paris 1926.
Vitztum: D. Vitztum, "Leprosy and lepers in Jerusalem" , *Teva V'aretz* 33/2 (1991) , pp. 38-41.
Volney: M.C.F. Volney, *Travels through Syria and Egypt in the Years 1783, 1784 and 1785*, London 1972.
Walton: A. Walton, *The Cult of Asklepios*, New-York 1965.
Wickersheimer: E. Wickersheimer, "Organisation et legislation sanitaires au Royaume franc de Jerusalem (1099–1291)", *Archives internationales d'histoire de Sciences*, 4 (1951), pp. 689–705.
Wilkinson: J. Wilkinson, *Jerusalem Pilgrims before the Crusades*, Jerusalem 1977.
William of Tyre: R.B.C. Huygens (ed.), *Guillaume de Tyr Chronique*, Corpvs Christianorum Continuatio Mediavalis, 63–63A, Turnhout 1986.
Woodings: A.F. Woodings, "The Medical Resources and Practice of the Crusader States in Syria and Palestine 1096–1193", *Medical History*, 15 (1971), pp. 268–277.
Ya'ari, Travels: A Ya'ari, *Travels in the Land of Israel*, (Ramat-Gan 1976).139. 1951. [H].
Ya'ari, Emissaries: A. Ya'ari, *Emissaries of the Land of Israel,* Jerusalem 1951. [H]
Ya'ari, Igrot: A. Ya'ari, *Igrot Eretz Israel [Letters of the Land of Israel*], Tel-Aviv 1943. [H]

Yadin, Scroll: Y. Yadin, *The Temple Scroll*, Tel-Aviv 1990.
Yadin: Y. Yadin, "Arabic Inscriptions in Palestine", *Eretz-Israel*, 7 (1964), pp. 102-116.
Yaniv: Z. Yaniv, "Medicinal plants through the generations", *Mada'* 26 (1) (1982) pp. 20-22. [H]
Yellin: D. Yellin, "Jewish Jerusalem of three hundred years ago", *Jerusalem ; Dedicated to A. M. Luncz*, Jerusalem 1928, pp. 78-105. [H]
Ze'evi: D. Ze'evi, An Ottoman Century: The District of Jerusalem in the Seventeenth Century, Jerusalem 1997. [H]
Zias, Garden: J.E. Zias "Garden of Eden or 'the house of isolation'?", *Teva Va'aretz* 29-6 (1987), pp. 17-19. [H]
Zias, Disease: J. E. Zias, Disease and healing methods in the ancient land of Israel in paleo-pathological research", *Qadmoniot,* 113 (1997) pp. 54-59. [H]
Zias, Lepers: J.E. Zias, "And they sent forth from the camp every leper and every person that has an issue", *Teva Va'aretz* 29 (1987), pp. 19-20. [H]
Zonta: M. Zonta, "Mineralogy, Botany and Zoology in Medieval Hebrew Encyclopaedias", *Arabic Sciences and Philosophy*, 6 (1996), pp. 263–315.

General Index

www.ingramcontent.com/pod-product-compliance
Lightning Source LLC
LaVergne TN
LVHW071213210926
848482LV00015B/802